Cementation in Dental Implantology

Chandur P.K. Wadhwani

Editor

Cementation in Dental Implantology

An Evidence-Based Guide

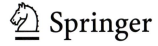 Springer

Editor
Chandur P.K. Wadhwani
University of Washington
School of Dentistry Restorative
Bellevue, WA
USA

ISBN 978-3-642-55162-8   ISBN 978-3-642-55163-5   (eBook)
DOI 10.1007/978-3-642-55163-5
Springer Heidelberg New York Dordrecht London

Library of Congress Control Number: 2014957637

Printed on acid-free paper

Springer is part of Springer Science+Business Media (www.springer.com)

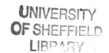

Acknowledgments

The authors wish to express their thanks to Jurijs Avots and Matt Barnard for their technical skills in fabricating the restorations shown in Chap. 7 (Figs. 7.1, 7.2, 7.3, 7.4, 7.5, 7.6, 7.7 7.37, 7.38, 7.39, 7.40, and 7.41). Also, thanks to Nakanishi Dental Laboratory for their scanning services shown in Chap. 4 (Fig. 4.37).

Contents

Contributors

Ken M. Akimoto, DDS, MSD Department of Periodontics, University of Washington, Private Practice Limited to Periodontics and Implant, Issaquah, WA, USA

Department of Periodontics, University of Washington School of Dentistry, Seattle, WA, USA

Curtis S.K. Chen, DDS, MSD, PhD Department of Oral Medicine, University of Washington, Seattle, WA, USA

Kwok-Hung (Albert) Chung, DDS, PhD Department of Restorative Dentistry, University of Washington School of Dentistry, Seattle, WA, USA

Tony Daher, DDS, MSEd Department of Restorative Dentistry, Loma Linda University, School of Dentistry, LaVerne, CA, USA

Private Practice Limited to Prosthodontics, LaVerne, CA, USA

Thomas Faber, DDS, MSD Department of Periodontics, University of Washington School of Dentistry, Seattle, WA, USA

Charles J. Goodacre, DDS, MSD Department of Restorative Dentistry, Loma Linda University School of Dentistry, Loma Linda, CA, USA

Kevin C. Lin, DDS Department of Integrated Reconstructive Dental Sciences, University of the Pacific, Arthur A. Dugoni School of Dentistry, San Francisco, CA, USA

Tomas Linkevičius, DDS, Dip Pros, PhD Department of Prosthetic Dentistry, Institute of Odontology, Vilnius University, Vilnius, Lithuania

Richard M. Opler, BA, DDS Senior Dental Student, University of Washington School of Dentistry, Seattle, WA, USA

Naomi Ramer, DDS Department of Pathology and Dentistry, Mount Sinai Hospital, New York, NY, USA

Neal Christopher Raval, BDS, MSD Private Practice Limited to Periodontics and Implant Dentistry, Bellevue, WA, USA

Ralf F. Schuler, Dr. Med. Dent, MSD Department of Periodontics, University of Washington School of Dentistry, Seattle, WA, USA

Private Practice Limited to Periodontics and Implant Dentistry, Seattle, WA, USA

Ernesto Ricardo Schwedhelm, DDS, MSD, FRCDC Department of Restorative Dentistry, University of Washington, School of Dentistry, Seattle, WA, USA

Private Practice Limited to Prosthodontics, Seattle, WA, USA

Diane Yoshinobu Tarica, DDS, FACP Private Practice Limited to Prosthodontics, Los Angeles, CA, USA

Chandur P.K. Wadhwani, BDS, MSD Department of Resotrative Dentistry, University of Washington School of Dentistry, Seattle, WA, USA

Private Practice Limted to Prosthodontics, Bellevue, WA, USA

Thomas G. Wilson Jr., DDS Private Practice Limited to Periodontics and Implant Dentistry, Dallas, TX, USA

Introduction

Clinical complications can occur with any dental treatment; dental implant therapy is no exception. It is important to know the types of problems that can occur with dental implants to develop an understanding of methods by which these can be minimized or, better yet, avoided altogether.

Complications associated with the cementation of crowns and fixed prostheses on dental implant abutments were first documented in the dental literature in the late 1990s. Since that time, scientific evidence and clinical experience have combined to propose methods of preventing unfavorable outcomes during cementation.

Dr. Wadhwani is a pioneer in examining the process of crown cementation on implant abutments. He is joined in this textbook by an exceptional group of scholars as chapter contributors, who add their special expertise to his research, and together there is an excellent synthesis of available evidence and clinical guidelines.

It is important that practitioners, educators, and students understand contemporary science regarding the cementation process associated with dental implants so complications can be reduced or eliminated. The profession will derive substantial benefit from this book that expands our knowledge and guides us to have a deeper understanding of how to optimize the cementation of crowns and fixed prostheses on implant abutments.

Charles J. Goodacre

The research and clinical material presented through the chapters was developed from a series of lectures and articles developed by the editor, Chandur Wadhwani, over the past 5 years.

The purpose of writing this book is to bring the clinicians involved in implant dentistry (surgeon and restorative) up to speed on what we have discovered related to the success and survival of dental implants. Implants can fail for many reasons; this book details one particular aspect that is believed to impact dental implant health: residual excess cement.

Apart from a large section dedicated to the issues associated with cement, there are sections on radiography and connection of implant components, all of which have relevance to the long success of dental implants. By informing the clinician of these issues, highlighting the difficulties, and providing some simple solutions, the problem can be more readily controlled and, hopefully, eliminated.

It is hoped that much of this material will be thought provoking and promote further study of this discipline with the overall goal of improving the value of these amazing medical devices (dental implants) that have changed the dental profession and improved the lives of countless patients.

The initial investigations were based on the need for a scientific approach to the restorative component of implant dentistry. At the time of completing this book, the editor/author has collaborated with over 30 researchers to help develop a series of protocols that can be applied in everyday practice. Much of this book has been developed from images and materials that were donated by esteemed clinicians who also offered advice and assistance, which cannot be overlooked. This book would not be possible if it were not for their unselfish sharing of information and their desire to find truth–all of which I believe will help advance the science of dentistry.

Chandur P.K. Wadhwani

These are a few of the many collaborators and researchers:

Ken Akimoto	Jurijs Avots	Jing Chen
Karim Alibhai	Matt Barnard	Tony Daher
Richard Ansong	Clark Chen	Richard Darveau
Daniel Asminovski	Curtis S. Chen	Thomas Faber
Fritz Finzen	Sylvia La Rosa	Paul Rosen
Stuart Froum	Kevin Lin	Ralf Schuler
Charlie Goodacre	Tomas Linkevičius	Ricardo Schwedhelm
Sabine Goodwin	Km Marshall	Arun Sharma
Dan Henry	David Nakanishi	Sang Tang
Dwight Hershman	Richard Opler	Diane Tarica
Timothy Hess	Kelli Palmer	Stuart Taylor
Steve Hurson	Avina Paranjpe	Anie Thomas
Sumita Jain	Alfonso Pineyro	Pilar Valderrama
James Johnson	Naomi Ramer	Tomas G. Wilson Jr.
Kevin Jones	Darrin Rapoport	Ryan Yousefian
Andrew Kim	Neal Raval	Hai Zhang
Stephanie Kretschmar	Danieli Rodrigues	

And especially my mentor and friend: Professor Kwok-Hung (Albert) Chung

Restoring the Dental Implant: The Biological Determinants

1

Chandur P.K. Wadhwani

Abstract

Dental implants should be considered as medical devices with an understanding that they behave in a very different way to the body part they replace—namely, the natural tooth. Implants have a soft tissue attachment mechanism to titanium that is a simple hemi-desmosomal cellular one; there is a lack of cementum so direct connective tissue fiber bundle attachment does not exist. The result is a system more vulnerable to insult from trauma than a healthy natural tooth.

Liabilities exist with implants that are not seen with the tooth, for example; commonly used techniques for teeth such as probing, retraction cord placement and cementation of a restoration, must be considered very differently. This chapter describes some of these issues with case reports.

Introduction

In the early 1980s, Branemark released information related to osseointegration and its experimental background. Out of the chance finding two decades earlier that titanium could be successfully integrated with bone was born the concept of osseointegration. From that moment, the world of dentistry would change forever. Tooth loss could now be predictably treated with dental implants and appropriate dental prostheses.

C.P.K. Wadhwani, BDS, MSD
Department of Restorative Dentistry, University of
Washington School of Dentistry, Seattle, WA, USA

Private Practice Limited to Prosthodontics,
1200, 116th Ave NE #A, Bellevue, WA 98004, USA
e-mail: cpkw@uw.edu

Today the concept of osseointegration is better understood than ever before, especially with the way that bone grows toward and against the surface of the dental implant. The bone provides the basis for retaining the implant within the human body, with mineralized tissue component firmly holding the titanium root form. Even after the implant is considered integrated, the cellular activity of the bone continues to develop by responding to the forces loaded upon it. Provided these forces are physiologically acceptable, the bone reacts by enhancing mineralization and further contributes to the improved stability of the implant.

From within the bony housing, the implant transcends through a soft tissue corridor and emerges into what is certainly the most hostile environment that exists within the human

C.P.K. Wadhwani (ed.), *Cementation in Dental Implantology: An Evidence-Based Guide,*
DOI 10.1007/978-3-642-55163-5_1, © Springer-Verlag Berlin Heidelberg 2015

body—the oral cavity. This environment is host to hundreds of microbial species with estimates of several billions of microbes present. The forces generated by the stomathological system and transmitted through the dentition are enormous, combined with the thermal (hot/cold) and chemical (acids/alkalis) insults of the diet. It is amazing that dental implants survive.

The soft tissue provides the implant with an initial protective barrier to prevent the ingress of bacteria and shield the implant from trauma. Knowledge of the cellular elements of the soft tissues at this site and how this heals over a short period of time is key to understanding the potential vulnerabilities that are present.

Soft Tissue Differences of Implants and the Natural Tooth

Comparing the soft tissue located around a tooth and an implant, there are some similarities, especially with the free gingival margin. In both cases, there exists buccal keratinized epithelium that extends into gingival sulcus where it transitions to become junctional epithelium. Apical to this is where the major differences occur.

A tooth crevice has keratinized epithelium at the base of the gingival sulcus, whereas an implant does not. The junctional epithelium of a tooth is adherent and less permeable and has a high capability to regenerate. An implant's epithelial attachment, by comparison, adheres poorly to the implant surface, is more permeable, and has a lower capacity to regenerate.

Apical to the junctional epithelium, along the surface of the implant, lies the soft connective tissue attachment. With a natural tooth, supracrestal connective tissue fiber bundles exist. These extend from the bone into the soft tissues, fanning out in multiple directions. Some extend from tooth to tooth in a horizontal manner, while others connect the soft tissues independently in a horizontal fashion and culminate in a mineralized attachment within living root cementum on the tooth root surface (Fig. 1.1). In health, the tooth to soft tissue connection system is considered a very robust mechanism that has evolved over mil-

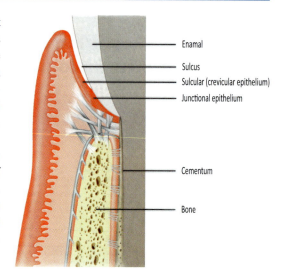

Fig. 1.1 The attachment mechanism of the natural tooth to the periodontal tissues. Note the fiber bundles' direction and how they connect to the tooth via the cementum (Reprinted from Rose LF et al. Periodontics: Medicine,Surgery and implants (2004). Copyright © 2004, with permission from Elsevier)

lions of years and serves as a seal to protect this area from insult.

With an implant, the attachment mechanism is more of a cellular adhesion to titanium, being hemi-desmosomal in nature. The implant site that develops through healing within a few days is far more fragile in comparison to the tooth connection; it tends to act more like a cuff and is considerably weaker. With implants, there are far fewer connective tissue collagen fiber bundles with no supracrestal fibers.

The fiber bundle direction is predominantly parallel or oblique to the implant surface. In a few instances, horizontal fibers have been described. However, these do not terminate onto mineralized living tissue, as there is no cementum on the implant surface (Fig. 1.2), and these horizontal fibers cannot be considered equivalent to those found associated with teeth, Sharpey's fibers.

One other major difference between the soft tissue attachment of the natural tooth and the implant is how the soft tissues allow for compartmentalization circumferentially. With the tooth, the fiber bundles attach at multiple sites to the cementum, producing distinct compartments that limit the progression of disease—consider the fiber bundles as being like spokes on a bicycle wheel. The segmentation produced by the fibers is noted by the disease processes that affect teeth such that periodontal disease is site specific. With an implant, essentially only one compartment exists, resulting from the circumferential fibers that encircle the implant, with disease here (peri-

implant disease) affecting the full 360° around the implant (Fig. 1.3a, b).

The consequences of the biological differences between the soft tissue attachments of teeth and implants can be readily demonstrated clinically as in the following three areas: disease pattern, probing effects, and displacement effects with retraction cord.

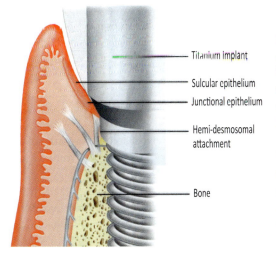

Fig. 1.2 The attachment of the soft tissue as the implant emerges through the body. The collagen fiber bundles run parallel or transverse to the implant long axis. One set of fibers encircles the implant like a "hula-hoop" (not shown). This attachment has taken only a few weeks to develop and is essentially a hemi-desmosomal connection (Reprinted from Rose LF et al. Periodontics: Medicine, Surgery and implants (2004). Copyright © 2004, with permission from Elsevier)

Disease Pattern: Biological and Clinical Significance— The Difference Between the Compartmentalization Seen with the Natural Tooth and That Seen Around an Implant

When periodontitis develops around a natural tooth, the bone changes tend to develop in a restrictive manner with distinct localized and angular defects noted. This is in stark contrast to the more generalized pattern of bone loss seen with periimplantitis, where crater- or well-type defects of bone loss circumvent the implant. The following case report describes this pattern:

Case Report #1

A 20-year-old female was referred to a periodontist for implant placement in the area of an existing mandibular right deciduous second molar, the permanent second bicuspid (tooth #29) having failed

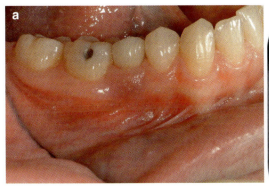

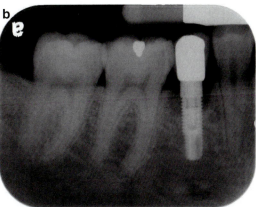

Fig. 1.3 (a, b) This implant site developed peri-implant disease. Initial soft tissue findings were cyanotic tissue that was inflamed. Radiographic examination shows the classic pattern noted with periimplantitis: circumferential bone loss with a crater-type bone defect

to develop. The site was evaluated for restorative and anatomical needs revealed by a cone beam computer tomogram with a radiographic guide in situ. An implant (Replace 3.5 mm diameter, 11.5 mm length; Nobel Biocare, USA) was placed by the periodontist according to the diagnostic criteria derived from the scan. The implant was allowed to heal for a period of 3 months and then was evaluated for both radiographic and clinical integrations. The patient returned to her restorative dentist for implant impressions, crown fabrication, and placement of the crown.

Two years' post-restoration, the patient represented at the periodontist's office with inflammation around the implant site, as shown in Fig. 1.3a, b.

The periodontist removed the crown and abutment and then removed the implant. On inspecting the implant, cement could be seen around the implant body with deposits of calculus on top (Fig. 1.4). The area was surgically debrided, and a bio-absorbable collagen wound dressing (CollaPlug, Zimmer Dental) was sutured across the surgical site. The area was left to heal for 3 months; then a crestal incision was made to retain the attached gingival and to expose the proposed implant site. The boney defect had filled in, although there was a slight residual buccolingual defect.

A new implant was placed along with a small amount of xenograft mineralized material (Bio-Oss, Osteohealth). The implant site was allowed to heal for 4 months; then the patient was sent to the restoring dentist for placement of a definitive crown, with instructions to use a screw-retained prosthesis.

Probing Differences Around Implants Versus Teeth: Biology and the Clinical Significance of the Soft Tissue Attachment—Differences In

To quantify the difference in these two attachments, a comparison of clinical probing forces can be made (see Fig. 1.5). The force advocated for probing around a natural, healthy tooth should be in the order of 0.25 N. In comparison, just over

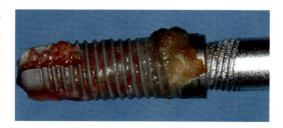

Fig. 1.4 The crown removed and implant removed by reverse torque. Calculus was noted on top of luting cement. This case is more completely described in chapter 11—Patterns Characteristic to Cement Induced-Peri-implant Disease (Reprinted with permission by *Dentistry Today* (Wadhwani and Pineyro 2012))

half this force around a healthy implant should be used—about 0.15 N.

The resistance to mechanical disruption of the two respective sites, a tooth and an implant, can be readily demonstrated with a diagrammatic representation of what occurs when the soft tissues are probed with the appropriate force (Fig. 1.5a, b). In the case of the healthy tooth, the robust nature of the fiber attachment is reflected in the manner the probe affects the tissues as well as the depth to which it extends. Compare this to a healthy implant attachment site where penetration is demonstrated, tearing away the hemidesmosomal connection.

Retraction Techniques: Biology and the Clinical Significance of the Soft Tissue Attachment

The use of a retraction cord as an isolation technique, as well as a physical barrier to cement extrusion beyond restorative finish lines, has been advocated, and while it may help prevent excess cement extrusion around healthy, natural teeth, it must be used with caution around implant restorations. The following case reports on the potential detrimental effects of placing a retraction cord around an implant abutment prior to cementing an implant crown.

Case Report #2

(From: Complications of using retraction cord protection of the peri-implant soft tissues against

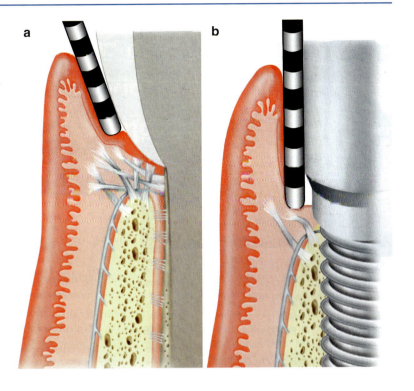

Fig. 1.5 (**a**, **b**) Probing: Implants versus teeth (Reprinted from Rose LF Periodontics:Medicine, Surgery and implants (2004). Copyright © 2004, with permission from Elsevier)

excess cement extrusion—A clinical report. Wadhwani and Ansong Reprinted with permission from Implant Realities 2012).

A 29-year-old healthy female patient was presented for implant restoration of the maxillary left lateral incisor. Six months earlier, an immediate implant (NobelReplace Select, Narrow platform, Nobel Biocare, Yorba Linda, CA, USA) had been surgically placed. This involved a traumatic removal of a retained fractured root remnant, followed by immediate implant placement. A buccal concavity existed on the facial aspect of the implant site; this was dealt with by raising a full-thickness mucogingival flap, placing a xenograft (NuOss, Ace Surgical Co., Inc., Brockton, MA, USA) for augmentation followed by a barrier membrane made of resorbable collagen (BioMend Extend, Zimmer, Carlsbad, CA, USA). The mucogingival flap was closed with sutures, and a 5-mm-tall healing abutment (Nobel Biocare) was placed onto the implant to allow soft tissue healing. Three months after the implant was placed, osseointegration was confirmed clinically by radiograph, as well as auscultation of the

implant. The healing cap was removed and a screw-retained acrylic provisional restoration made by using a temporary plastic abutment and a preformed acrylic crown. This was specifically designed to more closely match the soft tissue profile of a natural tooth. Following tissue maturation around the provisional abutment for a further 3 months, the implant was evaluated clinically and radiographically and considered ready for final restoration.

A custom impression coping was fabricated by modifying a stock impression coping by the addition of composite resin that mimicked the soft tissue contours around the implant. An impression was made using an open tray impression with an elastomeric impression material Express (3 M-ESPE, St. Paul MN, USA). A soft tissue gingival mask (Gingitech, Ivoclar-Vivadent, Amherst, NY, USA) was incorporated into a cast poured in type IV stone (Fuji Rock, GC, Leuven, Belgium) to provide the technician information on emergence profile, implant position, and depth, such that an implant abutment could be fabricated. The implant abutment was fabricated using computer-aided design/

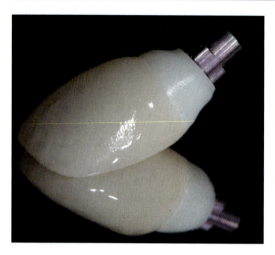

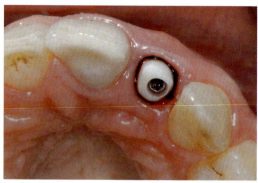

Fig. 1.7 The zirconium abutment in situ with retraction cord packed around the implant abutment, just apical to the restorative margin

Fig. 1.6 The zirconia abutment and crown, prior to placement. Note the color difference between the different materials necessitating subgingival margin placement

computer-aided manufacturing (CAD/CAM) by scanning with the Forte scanner (Nobel Biocare) and fabricating a milled zirconia abutment (Nobel Biocare), seen in Fig. 1.6.

For esthetic purposes, the zirconia abutment margin was placed 1 mm below the free gingival margin of the implant site. Once completed, the abutment was fixed to the implant analog within the cast and a crown was fabricated from Lava Ceram (3 M-ESPE, St. Paul, MN, USA). The restorative seating procedure consisted of removing the provisional crown to expose the implant platform. The abutment was oriented as designed, seated, and the abutment screw tightened to the appropriate torque (35 Ncm), as recommended by the manufacturer.

To reduce the effect of gingival fluid contamination, as well as to protect the tissues from excess cement extrusion, knitted retraction cord size 00 (Ultrapak, Ultradent Products Inc., South Jordan, UT, USA) was packed into the sulcus around the abutment. The retraction cord was measured to a length equivalent to the circumference of the abutment, cut, and then packed around the sulcus just apical to the abutment margin (Fig. 1.7).

After the crown was tried in, the esthetics and occlusion confirmed as acceptable to the patient and clinician, the intaglio of the crown was cleaned with phosphoric acid and washed in water, and then isopropyl alcohol was used as a saliva decontaminant. The adjacent teeth were isolated with PTFE tape (Oakley Co., Cleveland, OH, USA). The intaglio of the crown was loaded with cement (RelyX Unicem, 3 M-ESPE) and seated onto the abutment. Finger pressure was used to provide the crown seating force followed by light curing the facial cervical area for 10 s. Excess cement was removed with an explorer, followed by further light curing around and over the crown for 1 min. The subgingival retraction cord was located with a fine explorer, which, on removal, came out in multiple pieces with the cement remnants. Further cleanup of the cement margin was accomplished with hand instruments and dental floss. The fragmentation of the cord made measurement difficult; however, it appeared as though all of the cord was removed.

The patient was pleased with the esthetic result, the occlusion was checked, and the patient was dismissed. One week later, the patient presented with pain and erythema from the implant site (Fig. 1.8).

The area was also mildly fluctuant. The crown had been cemented with an adhesive cement which did not allow for the restoration to be removed without cutting it off. The crown was sectioned and removed.

On inspection of the gingival area adjacent to the abutment, a piece of cord was noted (Fig. 1.9a, b). This was removed, attached to which was a large mass of cement that had been extruded beyond the confines of the cord (Fig. 1.10a, b).

After complete debridement, the area was checked for any excess cement remnants. The provisional crown was reattached to the implant and the patient was dismissed. Two weeks later, the patient was reviewed and there were no clinical signs or symptoms related to the cement excess event. A new impression was made and a new abutment and crown fabricated. This time, the abutment margin was placed close to the free gingival margin, giving improved access to ensure complete removal of the cement lute.

Discussion

There is comparatively little research to guide practitioners on how to restore implants. Considering the vast numbers of implant systems and variations in products within companies, this may not be entirely surprising. However, in such

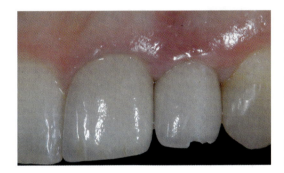

Fig. 1.8 One week after cementing the restoration. Erythema is noted on the peri-implant soft tissues; the crown is being cut to facilitate removal

an important area of dentistry, there is a need for more research on how to guide us on the most reliable restorations.

Retraction cord is frequently used as a means of expanding the sulcus around tooth preparations to expose a margin for impression making. It is also used as an isolation device to prevent gingival tissue fluid contamination of cements and helps reduce the excess cement extrusion during cementation of restorations on teeth. Although a useful tool, retraction cord use is not without issue, with injury due to mechanical as well as chemically impregnated cord, having been known for over half a century.

With the introduction of cementation procedures on implants, the problems associated with subgingival margins have been compounded. Excess cement extruded into the peri-implant tissues has been positively linked to peri-implant disease with numerous case reports documenting ill effects.

Material selection also presents with issues, for example, zirconia abutments have issues with predictable adhesion. The esthetics compound the issue, as the material is somewhat opaque and often dissimilar to that of the crown to be placed onto it. This requires a subgingival margin in esthetic sites, which has implications for cement.

The use of retraction cord as a means of isolating and protecting the soft tissues around an implant during cementation must be tempered against the fact that these tissues are substantially more fragile than those corresponding to a natural healthy attachment of a tooth.

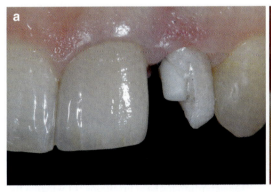
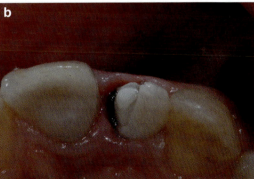

Fig. 1.9 (**a**) As the crown is removed, retraction cord is visible. (**b**) Occlusal view, demonstrating the cord remnants

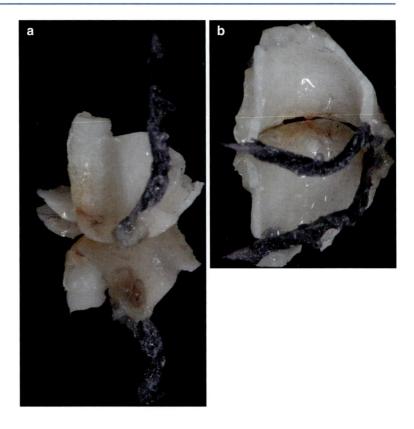

Fig. 1.10 (**a**, **b**) The cord is removed along with cement that has extruded beyond the area supposedly being protected. The outline shape of the implant is clearly visible

When considering the depth of the cemented margin with a tooth preparation, it is advisable to stay above the gingival sulcus where possible and, in esthetic sites, just beneath the free gingival margin. In contrast, implants are frequently placed 2–4 mm below the facial free gingival margin in esthetic sites. Where a natural tooth is adjacent to the implant, because of the tissue scalloping which rises at the papilla site, this may be 5–7 mm deep. This presents a significant difference again, which clearly places the peri-implant tissues at risk from insult with retraction cord.

Another factor that plays a role with the soft tissue vulnerability relates to the implant prosthetics, where manipulation of the soft tissue emergence profile to mimic the form of the root occurs. This is frequently achieved by tissue compression or displacement techniques resulting in blanched or tight tissues adjacent to the implant abutment. If this occurs, as in the case study reported, then the tight tissue must be further displaced to allow retraction cord access to the area below the margin of the abutment. This requires more force during cord placement, which inadvertently results in greater disruption of the fragile soft tissue attachment.

A review by Bennani et al, on the use of retraction cords with teeth and implants agreed that the displacement of implant soft tissues was very different to that of the tissues around a tooth. Clinicians should question the use of such procedures and the authors warned of the damage that may result from this procedure.

Another issue concerning the use of retraction cord is the fibrous nature of some cord materials. When a knitted cord is used with adhesive resin cement, it is likely that the cement will flow within the cord and adhere. Removal of the cord then becomes more challenging as it tends to stick or lock into place as the cement starts to set. If the cord tears and stretches (as noted in this case report), then on removal, it may give a false indication that it has been removed in its entirety, when in fact some remains in the sulcus.

One solution to these problems is to negate the use of cord by providing margins that are entirely above the free gingival margin, as documented in the implant crown with an esthetic adhesive margin described further in chapter 7. The ICEAM has porcelain margins that are amenable to hydrofluoric etching, silanation, and bonding. Margins above the free gingival tissues are esthetic with complete control of the cementation procedure, even if a highly adhesive resin is used, including cleanup. With restorations with less than ideal margin location, the clinician must consider this to be far more demanding. When undertaken, the use of a nonadhesive cement, for example, zinc oxide-eugenol, or zinc phosphate, or even eliminating the issue completely by fixing the restoration to the implant with a screw-retained restoration, should be considered.

Further Differences Between the Natural Dentition and the Dental Implant: How This Relates to Vulnerabilities Associated with Residual Excess Cement

Introduction

Understanding the differences biologically with the natural dentition and the implant must also include the challenges that present with both the site and environment in which they exist. All implants have susceptibilities to residual excess cement, some more than others due to their design features. Better understanding these differences can help the clinician minimize such risks.

Site Challenges

Indirect restorations placed on the natural tooth—for example, crowns—are usually planned such that the soft tissue depth of the cemented restoration is carefully controlled. The margins of some restorations must be extended slightly into the gingival sulcus 1/2–1 mm. The extension of any restorative margin into the gingival sulcus should be considered a compromise, but esthetic or retentive demands often make this necessary.

Careful control of this margin site is required. If this extends deeper below the tissues, it may infringe on the biological width, resulting in an inflammatory response. The impression making around tooth margins that are subgingivally placed also becomes more difficult. In general, the restorative dentist aims to prepare the natural tooth above the gingival margin and follow the contours of the soft tissue in a manner that provides for adequate restorative tooth length, does not damage the soft tissue, and allows for easy impression making. The result is usually an undulating finish line, raising at the papillae and supra-gingival at all low esthetic value sites.

The implant is very different. When placed according to soft tissue determinants, the implant surgeon is frequently requested to place the head (top) of the implant fixture 3 mm deep. If the implant lies adjacent to a tooth, the papillae sites may now be considerably deeper when compared to the facial areas. Sadan has suggested at interproximal sites that the distance from the tip of the papilla to the implant head could easily be 6–7 mm (Fig. 1.11).

The depth of the implant site potentially presents issues with both maintenance and microbial flora. Stambaugh reported on the inability for periodontal cleaning instrumentation to reach depths greater than 4 mm on the natural tooth, where the contours are usually less extreme when compared with the dental implant restoration.

Secondly, microbial flora that are considered etiological contributors to both periodontal and peri-implant diseases (the Gram-negative anaerobes) tend to favor deeper pocket sites. The depth of the implant and the microbial interaction with cements will be addressed in a later chapter.

Relating the depth of the implant, it should be noted that many of the latest implant systems no longer use the soft tissues as a starting site when planning the implant placement. Many use the bone reference markers now, with some implant systems advocating the head of the implant be placed 1–2 mm below the crest of the bone. This suggests that the implant placement is even deeper now and one can only assume the soft tissue depths adjacent to the implant are now 7 or more millimeters in depth (Fig. 1.12). This also

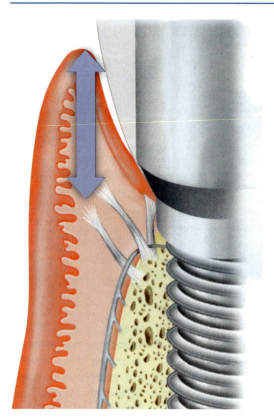

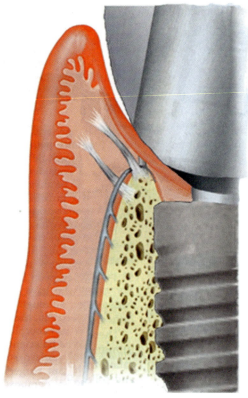

Fig. 1.11 If the head of the implant is placed 3 mm below the free gingival margin of the facial tissue, then where a papilla exists, this may extend to depths of 6–7 mm (Modified from: Rose LF et al. Periodontics: Medicine, Surgery and implants (2004))

Fig. 1.12 The bone crest is used as the reference for implant placement on the facial. This results in an increase of depth at the papilla site, which may be 8–9 mm deep (Modified from Rose LF et al. Periodontics: Medicine, Surgery and implants (2004))

highlights the issues with access to any residual excess cement (Figs. 1.13a, b and 1.14).

Several nuances are currently being explored with implant restorations. One such example is the use of a biologically active implant abutment. The company, BioHorizons, has designed an abutment to be placed in a bleeding soft tissue site, essentially an open wound (Fig. 1.15a, b). The concept is promoted as a healing response similar to that seen with an implant placement. If the implant has a rough surface to the top, a clot will initially form and adhere where blood contacts the implant. As the clot organizes, a fibrin attachment with the implant occurs. During further healing, the fibrin will contract toward the site where the clot had formed. The contraction tends to favor soft tissue healing in close proximity to the implant as well as providing a more

stable environment. Although this appears a reasonable idea on the implant body, the practicality of placing a roughened surface on the abutment must be considered carefully. During handling of the abutment components, a roughened surface on the underside of the implant abutment may be easily contaminated, especially if the soft tissues are not mature. During restoration if a temporary crown is cemented over the abutment as suggested by the manufacturer, any excess cement could easily extrude over the margin of the restoration and could flow into the rough implant abutment surfaces. Contamination of the roughened surface would not promote healing of the soft tissues and so would not result in the desired effect.

Implant abutment form also has a series of challenges that present to the clinician. For example, the contour is not always conducive to

Fig. 1.13 (**a**) An example of an implant placed deep within the tissues. The soft tissues between the implant and the bony socket must be considered for maintenance purposes. (**b**) This also highlights the difficulty in accessing excess cement. *Arrows* indicate excess cement sites

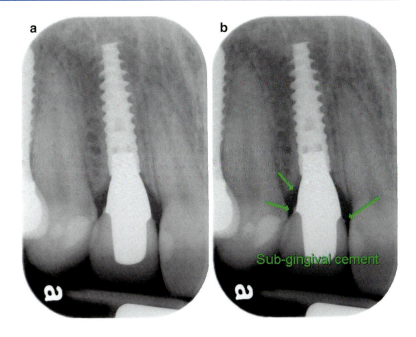

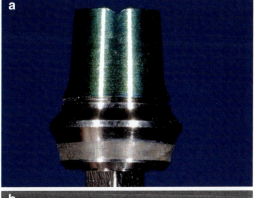

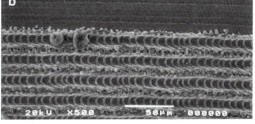

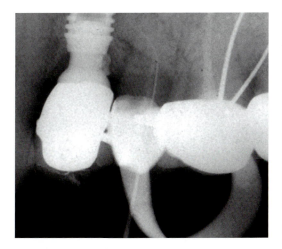

Fig. 1.14 A cemented restoration was placed on this implant. Residual excess cement can clearly be seen on the radiograph (Reprinted with permission by *Dentistry Today* (Muskiant 2010))

Fig. 1.15 (**a**, **b**) Some implant abutments are fabricated with a rough surface—with the expectation that blood clot maturation will allow tissue attachment (**a**). However, in practice, any contamination into this microscopic rough site (**b**) will interfere with healing, and removal of contaminating material such as cement is impossible

Fig. 1.16 (**a, b**) This platform-switched abutment shows that even without the restoration, it presents difficulty in accessing the residual excess cement with many of the instruments available today (Reprinted with permission by *Dentistry Today* (Wadhwani 2013))

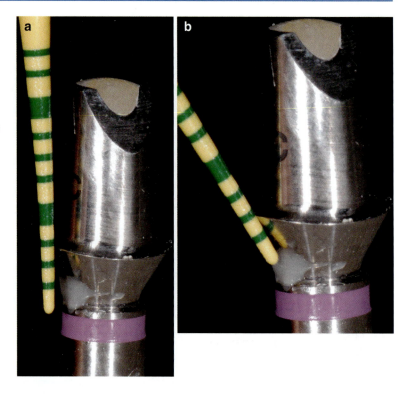

allowing access to cleansing or removal of excess cement (Fig. 1.16a, b). This example of a platform switching implant abutment clearly demonstrates the difficulty of gaining access to excess cement should it occur. The instrumentation currently available to most clinicians would not be capable of detecting excess cement, let alone removing it, if the event were to occur.

Other areas that provide challenges when considering adequate removal of access cement are the implants themselves. Some one-piece implants are contoured with an integral cement margin site that produces an undercut directly onto the implant body. This provides an environment that is very difficult to maintain when cement flows in and under this site, especially when the cement margin is close to this site (Fig. 1.17a–d).

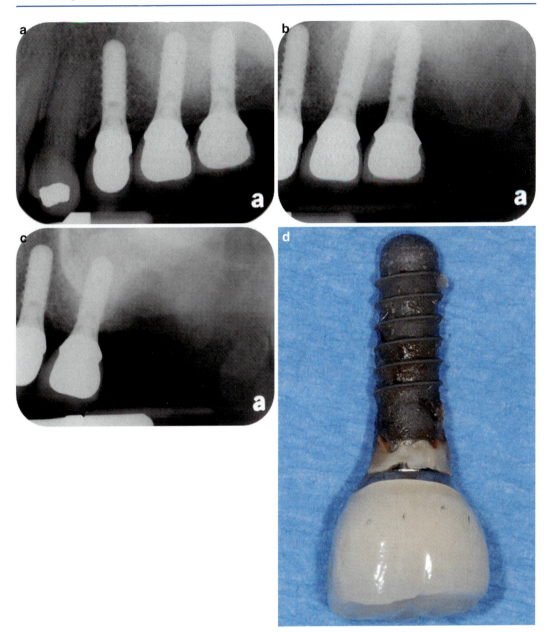

Fig. 1.17 (**a**) These 3 implants were restored in 2008; (**b**) 3 years later, routine radiograph indicates bone changes; (**c**) treatment of choice is implant removal. (**d**) The implant crown was cemented over a solid abutment. This does not allow for cement extrusion anywhere except at the margin of the crown which seats directly onto the implant. The contour is undercut and so cement will easily be expressed into this site, making cleanup very difficult pictures courtesy of Dr. Darrin Rapoport

Conclusion

The restorative implant dentist should have a good understanding of the challenges that go with placing and restoring these medical devices. Biological differences between a natural tooth and an implant, depth, and even shape of the implant all have a bearing on the problems being described. Most especially, the relative ease of disruption of the soft tissue connection associated with the implant must be taken into account to limit such damage, and the clinician must realize that commonly used practices on the natural tooth may not be applicable to the dental implant.

Bibliography

Akagawa Y, Takata T, Matsumoto T, Nikai H, Tsuru H. Correlation between clinical and histological evaluations of the peri-implant gingiva around the single-crystal sapphire endosseous implant. J Oral Rehabil. 1989;16:581–7.

Bartlett D. Implants for life? A critical review of implant-supported restorations. J Dent. 2007;35:768–72.

Bennani V, Schwass D, Chandler N. Gingival retraction techniques for implants versus teeth: current status. J Am Dent Assoc. 2008;139:1354–63.

Berglundh T, Lindhe J, Ericsson I, Marinello CP, Liljenberg B, Thomen P. The soft tissue barrier at implants and teeth. Clin Oral Implants Res. 1991;2:81–90.

Buser D, Weber HP. Soft tissue reactions to non-submerged unloaded titanium implants in beagle dogs. J Periodontol. 1992;63:225–35.

Callam D, Cobb C. Excess cement and peri-implant disease. J Implant Adv Clin Dent. 2009;1:61–8.

Ericsson I, Lindhe J. Probing depth at implants and teeth. An experimental study in the dog. J Clin Periodontol. 1993;20(9):623–7.

Gapski R, Neugeboren N, Pomeranz AZ, Reissner MW. Endosseous implant failure influenced by crown cementation: a clinical case report. Int J Oral Maxillofac Implants. 2008;23:943–6.

Gerber JA, Tan WC, Balmer TE, Salvi GE, Lan NP. Bleeding on probing and pocket probing depth in relation to probing pressure and mucosal health around oral implants. Clin Oral Implants Res. 2009;20:75–8.

Hansson HA, Albrektsson T, Brånemark P. Structural aspects of the interface between tissue and titanium implants. J Prosthet Dent. 1983;50:108–13.

Harrison JD. Effect of retraction materials on the gingival sulcus epithelium. J Prosthet Dent. 1961;11:514–21.

Hermann JS, Buser D, Schenk RK, Schoolfield JD, Cochran DL. Biologic width around one- and two-piece titanium implants. Clin Oral Implants Res. 2001;12:559–71.

James RA, Schultz RL. Hemidesmosomes and the adhesion of the junctional epithelial cells to metal implants—a preliminary report. Oral Implantol. 1974;4:294–302.

Löe H, Silness J. Tissue reactions to string packs used in fixed restorations. J Prosthet Dent. 1963;13:318–23.

Magne P, Belser U. Bonded porcelain restorations in the anterior dentition: a biometric approach. Carol Stream: Quintessence Publishing Co. Inc.; 2002.

Muskiant B. Ten hints for endodontic success. Dent Today. 2010;29(12):62.

Pauletto N, Lahiffe BJ, Walton JN. Complications associated with excess cement around crowns on osseointegrated implants: a clinical report. Int J Oral Maxillofac Implants. 1999;14:865–8.

Rose LF, Mealey BL, Genco RJ, Cohen WD. Periodontics, medicine, surgery and implants. Philadelphia: Elsevier Mosby; 2004. p. 612–3.

Sadan A, Blatz MB, Bellerino M, Block M. Prosthetic design considerations for anterior single-implant restorations. J Esthet Restor Dent. 2004;16:165–75.

Santos G, Santos M, Rizkalla A. Adhesive cementation of etchable ceramic esthetic restorations. J Can Dent Assoc. 2009;75:379–84.

Schroeder A, van der Zypen E, Stich H, Sutter F. The reactions of bone, connective tissue, and epithelium to endosteal implants with titanium-sprayed surfaces. J Maxillofac Surg. 1981;9:15–25.

Stambaugh RV, Dragoo M, Smith DM, Carasali L. The limits of subgingival scaling. Int J Periodontics Restorative Dent. 1981;1(15):30–41.

Stern IB. Current concepts of the dentogingival junction: the epithelial and connective tissue attachments to the tooth. J Periodontol. 1981;52:465–76.

Wadhwani CPK. The role of cements in dental implant success, part 1. Dent Today. 2013;32(4):76.

Wadhwani CP, Pineyro AF. Implant cementation: clinical problems and solutions. Dent Today. 2012;31:56. 58, 60–2.

Wadhwani CP, Pineyro A, Akimoto K. An introduction to the implant crown with an esthetic adhesive margin (ICEAM). J Esthet Restor Dent. 2012;27:246–54.

Wilson TG. The positive relationship between excess cement and peri-implant disease: a prospective clinical endoscopic study. J Periodontol. 2009;80: 1388–92.

Cemented Implant Restorations and the Risk of Peri-Implant Disease: Current Status

2

Chandur P.K. Wadhwani, Thomas G. Wilson Jr., and Kwok-Hung (Albert) Chung

Abstract

The relationship between implant disease and cement has evolved from multiple sources. Initially case studies, then a positive link, was established by Wilson. More evidence is presented by evaluating failed, removed implants and establishing if cement was present on the body of the implant. Although this does not explain why the peri-implant disease occurs, it does highlight significant problems dentists are having when restoring implants with cemented restorations.

Introduction

Dental implants have changed the way many dentists work and have improved the lives of countless patients. However, along with these positive changes have come some issues. One such example is the link between luting cements used for cement-retained implant restorations and peri-implant disease. How and why these materials cause an issue specifically with implants is currently under investigation. This chapter explores what we currently know about the interaction of cements, implants, and peri-implant diseases. The research and case reports presented here will hopefully provide an insight into the complexities of these disease processes. By providing a better understanding of what is occurring, it may be possible to reduce or even eliminate many of these problems.

The American Academy of Periodontology recently released a report reporting on peri-implant disease and risk factors.

The following are risk factors for peri-implant disease:

- Previous periodontal disease
- Poor plaque control/inability to clean
- Residual cement
- Smoking
- Diabetes
- Occlusal overload
- Potential emerging risk factors (alcohol, rheumatoid arthritis, loading too late)

C.P.K. Wadhwani, BDS, MSD (⊠)
Department of Restorative Dentistry,
University of Washington, Seattle, WA, USA

Private Practice Limited to Prosthodontics,
1200, 116th Ave NE #A, Bellevue, WA 98004, USA
e-mail: cpkw@uw.edu

T.G. WilsonJr. , DDS
Private Practice Limited to Periodontics and Implant
Dentistry, Dallas, TX, USA

K.-H. (Albert) Chung, DDS, PhD
Department of Restorative Dentistry,
University of Washington School of Dentistry,
Seattle, WA, USA

C.P.K. Wadhwani (ed.), *Cementation in Dental Implantology: An Evidence-Based Guide*,
DOI 10.1007/978-3-642-55163-5_2, © Springer-Verlag Berlin Heidelberg 2015

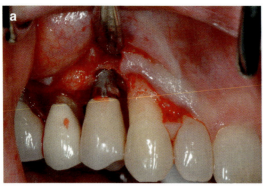
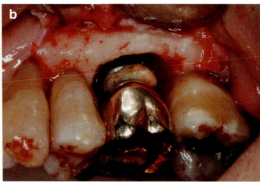
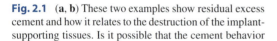

Fig. 2.1 (**a**, **b**) These two examples show residual excess cement and how it relates to the destruction of the implant-supporting tissues. Is it possible that the cement behavior was active in this process, or did it simply occur because the cement presented an overhang of material?

When the list is critically reviewed, it is clear that some of these risk factors are within the control of the restorative dentist, especially providing a reconstruction that is accessible to cleansing adequately, and more importantly, the complete elimination of residual excess cement when a cement-retained restoration is used.

Cement-retained restorations for implants were introduced over 20 years ago, with many claimed advantageous such as control of esthetics, occlusion, cost, ease of fabrication, and passive fit. However, it is more likely that this type of restoration became popular because dentists were familiar with the cementation process, it being a part of traditional tooth form dentistry. What is of interest to note is that most patients, when surveyed, do not mind whether they receive a screw- or cement-retained restoration; therefore, it appears to be predominately the clinician's choice to use a cement-retained restoration.

Controversies exist about this disease process, and the aim of this chapter is to explore what is currently known about peri-implant disease and question why implants are so susceptible to a process dentistry has been using for over 100 years with great success vis-à-vis cementing restorations onto natural teeth. Peri-implant disease is now considered to be comprised of two general categories: peri-implant mucositis and periimplantitis. Some authorities consider peri-implant mucositis to be similar in nature to gingivitis, in that it is restricted to the soft implant-supporting tissues and is considered reversible if treated early. In contrast, periimplantitis is a irreversible disease process that affects the supporting bone tissues, and, although considered similar to periodontitis, it is noted to be far more aggressive and difficult to control.

Although the peri-implant disease process has several risk factors, where residual excess cement is concerned, it may be that the cement has an active etiological role rather than simply behaving as a mechanical trap for bacteria such as an overhang (Fig. 2.1a, b). Peri-implant disease may be promoted by the presence of residual excess cement due to bacterial interaction, allergic response, foreign body reaction to cement, or by the cement altering the surface of the implant resulting in inflammation around the site.

The Science and Studies—Microbial Interaction: T.G. Wilson's Study on the Clinical Relationship Between Residual Excess Cement and Peri-implant Disease

By definition, peri-implant diseases are inflammatory in nature. Many of the same pathogenic bacteria associated with periodontal diseases are also associated with peri-implant disease. Several case reports found these inflammatory lesions (peri-implant mucositis and periimplantitis) were associated with residual cement.

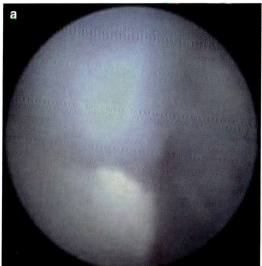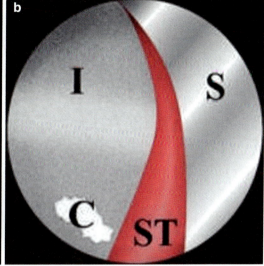

Fig. 2.2 (**a**) A piece of cement, 0.5 mm in diameter, attached to the implant surface is seen in the lower left quadrant of the screen grab from the endoscope. (**b**) An illustration of A. *I* implant, *S* shield, *C* cement, *ST* soft tissue (Reproduced with permission from the American Academy of Periodontology: Wilson (2009))

A prospective inception cohort study on the relationship of excess cement to peri-implant disease was published in 2009. A dental endoscope was employed to view the subgingival peri-implant space. Inflammation around fixtures was often found associated with dental cement adhering to the implant superstructure or to the fixture its superstructure.

Individuals presenting with clinical signs of peri-implant mucositis (bleeding upon probing, color change) had the peri-implant space debrided and their oral hygiene reinforced and were instructed to irrigate the affected area with chlorhexidine 0.12 % twice daily for 30 days. If bleeding or other signs of clinical inflammation were still present 30 days later, the patient was entered into the study. Patients who presented with suppuration, had increased probing depths, or had radiographic evidence of continued bone loss were entered directly into the study. Thirty-nine consecutive patients with 42 implants were entered. Twelve of these patients had 20 similar implants that had no signs of peri-implant disease. These last implants served as controls. All test and control implants had received cemented single-unit fixed partial dentures. Both groups had the subgingival peri-implant site explored using a dental endoscope (Fig. 2.2a, b).

The presence or absence of materials adherent to the implant itself, the crown, and any material visualized in the surrounding soft tissues was recorded. This generation of endoscope dental cement has a brilliant white reflectivity; calculus is dull brown and biofilm gray/blue. Biofilm can be easily removed with the tip of the endoscopic explorer. Removal of any adherent material was accomplished using the scope for visualization and combinations of hand and/or mechanical methods until no further material could be visualized. The endoscope explorer was then rotated 180°, and any materials visualized in the soft tissues were removed, if possible (Fig. 2.3a, b).

Cement was found on 81 % of the test implants and on none of the control fixtures. At the 1-month evaluation, after removal of foreign matter, 76 % of the clinical and endoscopic signs of inflammation around the test implants had resolved. Three of the test implants required surgical entries to resolve the inflammatory process. Studies of biopsies from these three cases, as well as a number of additional cases, are currently underway.

One of the most disturbing aspects of this data was that the earliest signs of peri-implant disease

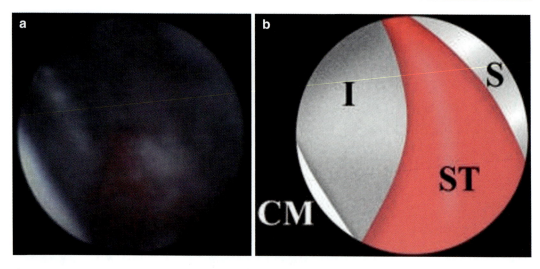

Fig. 2.3 (**a**) An endoscopic view of the same implant seen in Fig. 2.1 after cement removal. (**b**) An illustration of (**a**). *I* implant, *S* shield, *CM* crown margin, *ST* soft tissue (Reproduced with permission from the American Academy of Periodontology: Wilson (2009))

did not appear until 4 months after cementation, while the longest was 9 1/2 years after placement (Fig. 2.4). The findings of this study have been duplicated by others.

While in this study the type of cement used did not appear to affect the disease process, recent evidence suggests that some cement types may have an active role in the disease process.

As a result of the cumulative information available, so far it appears that modifying surgical and prosthetic approaches when using cemented crowns are important. Prosthetic modifications and the use of alternative types of cement are addressed in other chapters of this book.

Surgical modifications include reduction of excess soft tissues, which may interfere with cement removal, flattening posterior ridges to eliminate redundant soft tissue, the use of implants with smooth gingival collars designed to raise the crown/implant margin coronal to the soft tissues, and placing the coronal portion of the implant as shallow as possible, while keeping esthetic and functional aspects in mind.

Treating implants that have lost bone attachment as a result of periimplantitis remains problematical. At present, the only proven way to stop the progress of periimplantitis is to remove the rough surface of the implant. This presents obvious esthetic and food impaction problems. One of the keys to achieving new bony attachment on an implant surface previously covered by biofilm is the successful removal of the bacteria and their byproducts. While many approaches have been tried, the final answer is not yet available. One technological advance, the video scope, allows increased visualization and a greater potential to remove implant-borne and soft tissue-associated particles. These particles are frequently found to be cement and titanium. Studies on their role in the etiology of peri-implant diseases, as well as the treatment of these diseases, continue.

At present, it is important to educate dental professionals about the problem and to periodically evaluate the peri-implant tissues monitoring for early indications of disease. When peri-implant mucositis is detected early, treatment should be

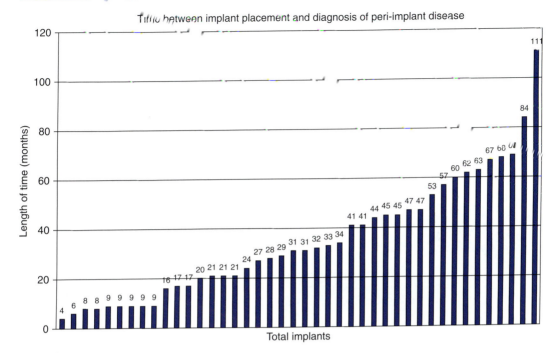

Fig. 2.4 The presence of peri-implant disease was discovered as soon as 4 months after cementing the fixed partial denture and as long as 111 months. Each bar represents an individual implant (Mean 2.93 years) (Reproduced with permission from the American Academy of Periodontology: Wilson (2009, 1390))

immediately employed to prevent this evolving into periimplantitis with associated bone loss.

Case Reports Where Residual Cement Was Associated with Peri-implant Disease

Figure 2.5a shows a female patient who presented with cervical resorption of the maxillary right canine with symptoms of irreversible pulpitis. Radiograph is shown in Fig. 2.5b. Treatment of choice was extraction and implant placement.

Post extraction, the surgical site was carefully evaluated and bone thickness recorded. This was considered appropriate for immediate implant placement (Implant: Nobel Biocare

Replace). Figure 2.5(c-d) Radiographic imaging showed the implant to be in a good position, the soft tissue was supported by the use of allograft particulate material (Bio-Oss, Giestlich). To prtects and support the soft tissues further a custom healing abutment was fabricated Figure 2.5e. The implant was left to integrate for 3 months prior to referral back to the restoring clinician.

Three years after implant restoration was completed, the patient represented at the periodontist's office complaining of pain. Figure 2.6a the clinical photograph; note the tissue changes mesial to the implant site. The Radiograph (Fig. 2.6b) indicated bone loss. Full-thickness soft tissue flap elevation revealed the extent of this lesion (Fig. 2.6c). In Fig. 2.6d, the cement

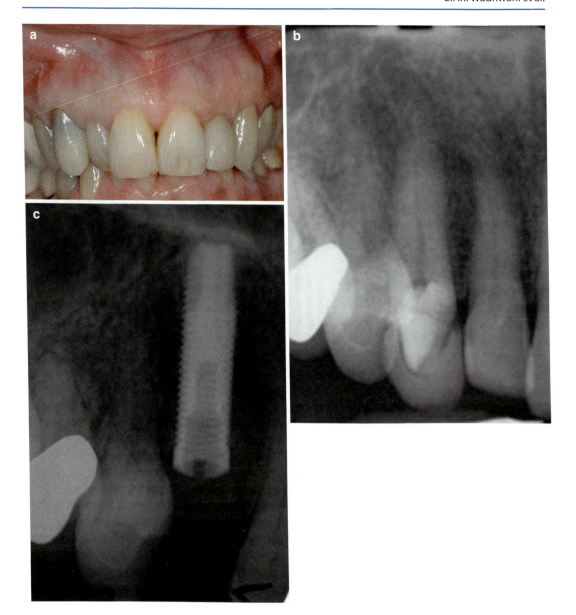

Fig. 2.5 (**a**) This female patient presented with cervical resorption of the maxillary right canine with symptoms of irreversible pulpitis. (**b**) Radiograph is shown. Treatment of choice was extraction and implant placement. (**c–e**) Post extraction, the surgical site was carefully evaluated and bone thickness recorded. This was considered appropriate for immediate implant placement (Implant: Nobel Biocare Replace). (**c**) Radiograph showing implant placed. (**d**) Cervical area augments with allograft particulate matter (Bio-Oss). (**e**) Custom healing abutment being fabricated, using a temporary plastic cylinder. This was provided to maintain the soft tissue profile during the healing phase. The implant was left to integrate for 3 months prior to referral back to the restoring clinician

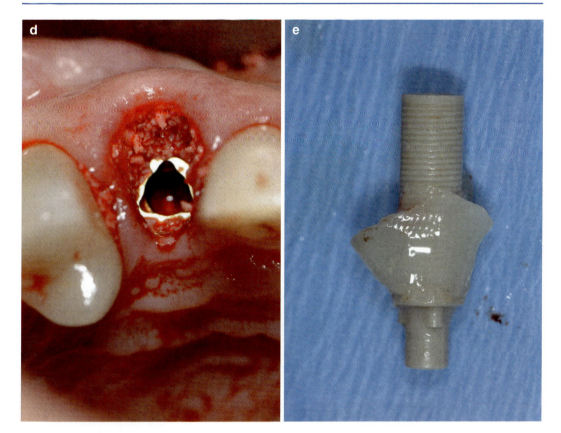

Fig. 2.5 (continued)

is clearly visible. This case and the associated treatment outcome is described further in chapter 11.

Prevalence of the Cement-Induced Peri-implant Disease Issue

Thomas Wilson is credited with being the first investigator to describe the link between residual excess cement and peri-implant disease. To date no data exists on how many implants fail that may be the result of an interaction with cement extrusion. Even if cement is not the direct cause of implant loss, it would be of value to determine how frequently it is found associated with implants that fail.

In August 2011, Nobel Biocare, USA, allowed a sample of returned failed implants over a 6-week period to be evaluated. The implants and associated information (patient data, date placed, date failed, potential failure causes, etc.) were recorded. The implants with their restorations were photographed, and any material attached to the implant or abutment was subject to energy dispersive spectroscopy (EDS). This allows a nondestructive identification of foreign material adhesions to the surface of failed and returned implants that were inspected for materials attached (Figs. 2.7, 2.8, 2.9, 2.10, 2.11, 2.12, and 2.13).

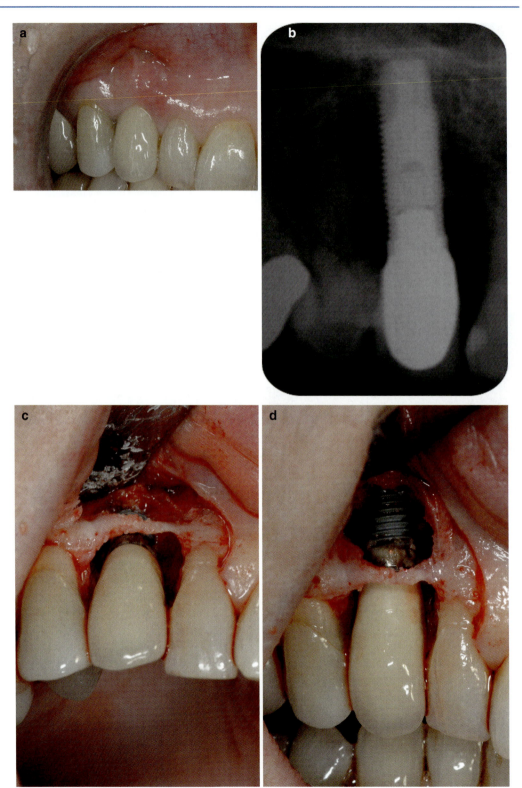

Fig. 2.6 (**a–d**) Three years after implant restoration, the patient re-presented at the periodontist's office complaining of pain. (**a**) Clinical photograph, note tissue changes mesial to the implant site. (**b**) Radiograph indicates bone loss. (**c**) Full-thickness soft tissue flap elevation shows the extent of this lesion. (**d**) The cement is clearly visible

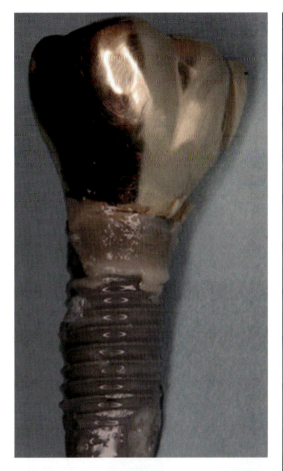

Fig. 2.7 Example of a failed implant with residual excess cement. XRF analysis determined this as RelyX luting cement

Data Collection Technique and Results

Elemental analysis of materials is useful in many scientific disciplines, providing quantitative and qualitative data on the elemental composition of materials. However, this often results in destruction of the specimen being tested, which in some fields is highly undesirable. Medical X-ray fluorescence spectroscopy (XRF) provides a nondestructive means of estimating elemental composition in humans and has been used in research for in vitro and in vivo for many years. The XRF instrument uses low-level gamma radiation to provoke the emission of fluorescent photons from the target area being tested. The photons are detected and counted over the wave-

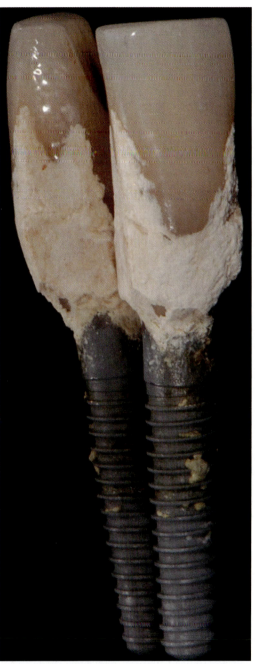

Fig. 2.8 This failed implant (with mirror) had a note from the surgeon stating the patient was a smoker and that may have contributed to the implant failure. The material was examined and determined to be calculus on top of a resin-based cement

length spectrum from which characteristic emission patterns unique to each element may be recorded. The XRF machine can be used for

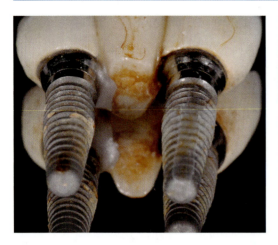

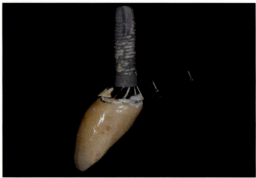

Fig. 2.11 Cement is clearly visible at the margin of this specimen. It also extended halfway down the implant. The other materials noted were bone mineral deposits extending to the full length of the implant

Fig. 2.9 Failed implant bridge after 8 years of service. The implant documentation stated the implants were placed in October 2001, restored in April 2002, and removed in May 2010

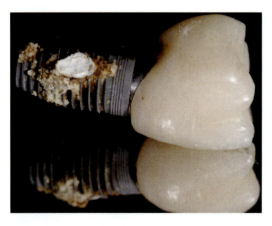

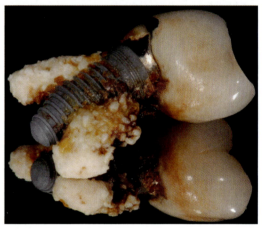

Fig. 2.10 Another failed implant with residual excess cement noted all the way down onto the screw threads. It should be stated that cement may not be the cause of failure in some cases; however, the lack of control of the clinician with the cementing technique is clear

Fig. 2.12 This example had cement, calculus, and bone mineral deposits the full length of the implant body. The size of defect on removal of this failed implant is unimaginable!

varying degrees of material penetration, which affects the level of electron shell emission. Weaker penetrating X-rays are usually used for non-mineralized tissues and have been used in vivo to investigate tissue structures such as the eye, skin, prostate, kidney, liver, thyroid, spleen, and lungs. For mineralized materials, such as bone, where deeper penetration of the X-rays is desired, the K-shell ($K\alpha$) emissions are considered more useful.

Identification of materials used in dentistry is also important, especially when the material has an adverse effect on the surrounding tissue. One such example that has recently come to light is the detection of residual cement material extruded at the crown margin, used for cement-retained implant restorations. A positive link has been established between excess cement extrusion and peri-implant disease, identified with an endoscopic device. Excess cement can also be detected radiographically, given the cement is radiopaque enough: described in chapter 5. One problem is confirming the material tested if it is in fact dental cement and not mineral deposits such as calculus

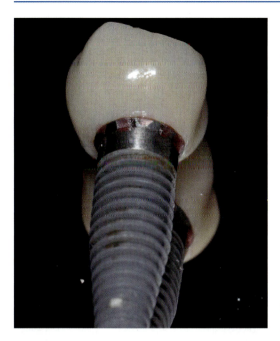

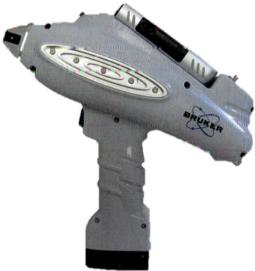

Fig. 2.14 The Bruker TRACeR III-V X-ray fluorescence analyzer (Photo courtesy of Bruker Elemental, Kennewick, WA, USA)

Fig. 2.13 Some cements could be clearly identified by their physical characteristics; this pink cement was Premier implant cement

or bone. If the cement can be removed, it may be further analyzed using a variety of techniques including visual, light microscope, and SEM or even subject to elemental analysis using traditional methods such as mass spectroscopy. However, many of these methods require the sample be modified or degraded and are time consuming and costly. Some also require that the specimen be destroyed.

The need to evaluate foreign materials on the surface of dental implants may provide clues as to the understanding of how and why implants fail. Here we describe a simple nondestructive technique for the identification of residual foreign material attached at the margin of a cement-retained implant restoration or on the surface of the body of the implant.

Procedure

A handheld wide-range elemental analyzer (TRACeR III-V; Bruker AXS Inc., Madison, Wisc) (Fig. 2.14) connected to a personal com-

puter running the Bruker S1PXRF software was used. The instrument was based on energy dispersive X-ray fluorescence (XRF) technology and contains a high-resolution, thermoelectric cooling, silicon PIN (Si-PIN) diode detector. As this device can identify the elemental makeup of a product, it was necessary to have sample cements evaluated for their elemental spectra. To create the reference spectrums, six commonly used cements were mixed according to the manufacturers' instruction (Table 2.1) and used to fabricate the disc specimens as a control for calculus, and human bone was also tested. As a control, spectrums of deposits removed from cervical regions of lower anterior teeth are known to be calculus, and bone fragments removed from extraction sites of human teeth are also created. All specimens were autoclave sterilized prior to XRF analysis. Each specimen was placed over the aperture of the machine and exposed for 60 sec at 40 kV and 20 μA. The resultant fluorescence data, recorded as intensity counts, was displayed in spectral form on the computer. Elements in the spectra data were identified using the predefined major peaks (Kα or Lα) of the S1PXRF program.

The failed implants with excess foreign material around the implant surface were placed in the

Table 2.1 Major peaks of spectra of commonly used cements, bone, and calculus

Material	Major peaks	Examples
ZnO-type cement	ZnKα1	TempBond NE, IRM
Glass ionomer cement	SrKα1, ZrKα1	RelyX Unicem
Polycarboxylate cement	SrKα1, SnKα1	Duralon
Resin cement	No major peak	PIC[a]
Alveolar bone	CaKα1	–
Dental calculus	CaKα1	–

TempBond NE – Kerr Corp; IRM – Dentsply Caulk; RelyX Unicem – 3 M ESPE; Duralon – 3 M ESPE
[a]PIC– Premier Implant cement, Premier Products Co, Plymouth, Pennsylvania

XRF evaluation chamber on the aperture and analyzed with the same parameter used for the controls. With the implant body partially overlying the aperture, a peak for the element titanium was expected as well as peaks for the attached test material. The XRF also quantifies elements within the test area, with the largest elemental peak height representing the most abundant element. The peaks of the unknown sample spectrum were identified and labeled using the "ID" and "Elem" tools of the S1PERF program. The Bruker has a spectrum overlay function which allows superimposition of a known material with a test material for comparison. The spectra of the unknown sample was put in the background in red and the reference spectra derived from known composition of the samples (cement, calculus, and bone) overlaid.

In total, 189 implants were examined with the spectrometer. Sixty-five percent had cement extrusion remnants found on the major screw threads of the implant. Although it is not possible to state to what extent the cement extrusion played in the role of these implant failures, it is clear that the cementing technique of the operators leaves much to be desired; the cement should be controlled so as never to extrude beyond the cement margins.

Conclusion

Residual excess cement has been positively linked in clinical studies with peri-implant disease. The identification of material on the implant body itself does not explain how this disease process develops and is not conclusive of a cause/effect relationship. It does, however, still validate how the cementing techniques widely used in restoring implants are poorly controlled. The depth the cement reached indicated in the failed implant study is also of great concern.

Bibliography

American Academy of Periodontology. Peri-implant mucositis and peri-implantitis: a current understanding of their diagnoses and clinical implications. J Periodontol. 2013;84:436–643.

Borjesson J, Mattsson S. Medical applications of X-ray fluorescence for trace element research. ICDD Data; 2007. ISSN 1097-0002.

Callam D, Cobb C. Excess cement and peri-implant disease. J Implant Adv Clin Dent. 2009;1:61–8.

Gapski R, Neugeboren N, Pomeranz AZ, Reissner MW. Endosseous implant failure influenced by crown cementation: a clinical case report. Int J Oral Maxillofac Implants. 2008;23:943.

Hu H, Aro A, Rotnitzky A. Bone lead measured by x-ray fluorescence: epidemiological methods. Environ Health Perspect. 1995;103:105–10.

Jung R, Zembic A, Pjetursson BE, Zwahlen MS, Thoma D. Systematic review of the survival rate and the incidence of biological, technical, and aesthetic complications of single crowns on implants reported in longitudinal studies with a mean follow-up of 5 years. Clin Oral Implants Res. 2012;23(s6):2–21.

Mombelli A, Müller N, Cionca N. The epidemiology of peri-implantitis. Clin Oral Implants Res. 2012;23(6):67–76.

Pauletto N, Lahiffe BJ, Walton JN. Complications associated with excess cement around crowns on osseointegrated implants: a clinical report. Int J Oral Maxillofac Implants. 1999;14:865–8.

Tarica DY, Alvarado VM, Truong ST. Survey of United States dental schools on cementation protocols for implant crown restorations. J Prosthet Dent. 2010; 103:68–79.

Taylor T, Agar JR. Twenty years of progress in implant prosthodontics. J Prosthet Dent. 2002;88:89–95.

Valderrama P, Wilson Jr TG. Detoxification of implant surfaces affected by peri-implant disease: an overview of surgical methods. Int J Dent. 2013;1:1–9.

Wadhwani C, Rapoport D, La Rosa S, Hess T, Kretschmar S. Radiographic detection and characteristic patterns of residual excess cement associated with cement retained implant restorations: a clinical report. J Prosthet Dent. 2012;107:151–7.

Webber HP, Kim DM, Ng MW, Hwang JW, Fiorellini JP. Peri-implant soft-tissue health surrounding cement- and screw-retained implant restorations: a multi-center, 3 year prospective study. Clin Oral Implants Res. 2006;17:375–9.

Wilson TG. The positive relationship between excess cement and peri-implant disease: a prospective clinical endoscopic study. J Periodontol. 2009;80:1388–92.

Peri-implant Disease and Cemented Implant Restorations: A Multifactorial Etiology

3

Chandur P.K. Wadhwani, Neal Christopher Raval, and Naomi Ramer

Abstract

The etiological factors related to peri-implant disease have yet to be fully understood. In the case of cement-induced issues, several theories have been developed ranging from microbial colonization of cements, giant cell reaction, allergic response and activation of titanium. This chapter explores some of these factors, through research and examination. It may be that some or all of the disease entities may come from an overt immune response precipitated by these factors working alone or in combination.

Introduction

Dental implants should be considered as highly sophisticated medical devices. As such, they provide real value to our patients and have the ability to improve quality of life. With the introduction of the cemented restoration came the ability to restore the implant in a manner similar to how we deal with the natural dentition, namely, crown and bridge prosthetics. However, over the past few years, there appears to be an increase in the incidence of peri-implant disease that may be associated in one form or another with this type of restoration.

This chapter introduces some unique studies undertaken by the authors which may help explain some of the complexities related to the etiology of cement-induced peri-implant disease.

A recent report by the American Academy of Periodontology now includes residual cement as a risk factor for peri-implant disease (per-implant mucositis and peri-implantitis). It would appear that all implants are potentially susceptible to peri-implant disease (Fig. 3.1a–c). The purpose of this chapter is to explore why such a relationship between cements, implants, and disease may exist and give guidance related to prevention of this problem.

A common misconception is that it is only the type of luting cement used that either results in an

C.P.K. Wadhwani, BDS, MSD (✉)
Department of Restorative Dentistry, University of Washington dental School,
Seattle, WA, USA

Private Practice Limited to Prosthodontics,
1200, 116th Ave NE #A, Bellevue, WA 98004, USA
e-mail: cpkw@uw.edu

N.C. Raval, BDS, MSD
Private Practice Limited to Periodontics
and Implants, Bellevue, WA, USA

N. Ramer, DDS
Department of Pathology and Dentistry, Oral and
Maxillofacial Pathology Residency Program,
Mount Sinai Hospital, New York, NY, USA

C.P.K. Wadhwani (ed.), *Cementation in Dental Implantology: An Evidence-Based Guide*,
DOI 10.1007/978-3-642-55163-5_3, © Springer-Verlag Berlin Heidelberg 2015

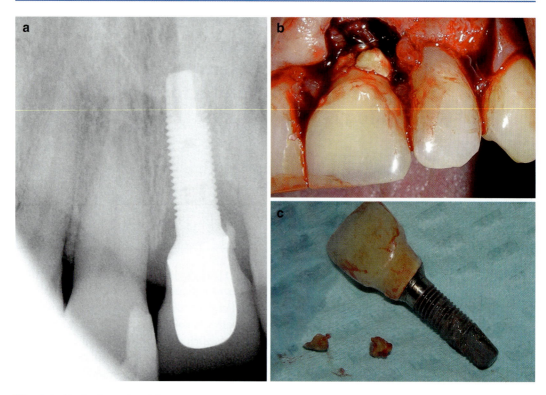

Fig. 3.1 (**a**) Radiograph of implant and associated cement. (**b**) Clinical picture after surgical flap elevation. Cement on the surface of an implant with extensive bone loss associated with this disease. (**c**) Implant is removed with cement residue

implant disease process or not. Any cement can lead to destruction around an implant, although in truth some cements may have more issues than others; the disease process, like most diseases, is multifactorial.

Factors such as understanding why implants are vulnerable to cement-induced disease process due to biology, depth, environment, implant materials, cement properties, cement application, abutment design, and maintenance are all important if peri-implant diseases are to be prevented.

Dentists are familiar with dealing with the natural dentition and as such have taken many of the concepts and techniques used when restoring a tooth with a cemented restoration and transferred them to the cemented implant restoration. This must be considered an error. Teeth and implants have very different requirements with respect to how the tissues attach, the depth of margin placement, the disease susceptibility, and the core materials of the abutment (enamel and dentine for the tooth versus ceramics, zirconia, or metal for the implant; Figs. 3.2 and 3.3a–c).

Current Understanding of Peri-implant Disease and Residual Excess Cement: Etiology

It is unclear why the cement should cause an issue, as well as to what role the cement plays in this process. It is possible that the cement is simply passive and acts as a physical bacterial trap, rather like an overhang on a restoration or calculus effects on the natural dentition (Fig. 3.4). It is also possible that the cement plays more of an active role, as the destruction of the peri-implant tissues (hard and soft) is frequently aggressive and extensive (Fig. 3.5a, b). The disease may be different between patients, and even within the same patient. It may be due primarily to one major factor or a combination of factors (Figs. 3.6, 3.7, and 3.8a, b).

There are currently four potential causes of peri-implant disease as it relates to residual cement: microbiology, foreign body reaction, allergic response, and alterations in implant surfaces.

Microbiological

Wilson suggested that the disease process he noted may be microbiological in nature. This was in part due to the time it took for signs and symptoms to develop. This ranged from 4 months to 9.3 years after the cement-retained implant restoration was placed.

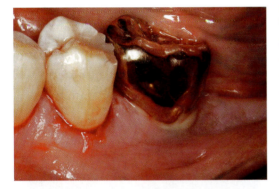

Fig. 3.2 This case shows the effects of residual excess cement resulting in peri-implant disease with suppuration a common finding

Certainly the environment around implants is conducive to Gram-negative pathogenic bacteria. Depths of 5–7 mm adjacent to a papilla provide anaerobic sites that allow for their potential growth. Although much has been reported on physical and chemical properties of cements, there appears to be nothing related to how cements interact with sites that may harbor these bacteria. An ongoing research project the author is involved with at the University of Washington has recorded variations in the growth patterns of media containing *Aggregatibacter actinomycetemcomitans* (Aa), *Fusobacterium nucleatum* (Fn), and *Porphyromonas gingivalis* (Pg) when exposed to different cements.

The study involved the University's graduate periodontal and microbiology departments and formed the basis of Dr. Neal Raval's Master's thesis. To the authors' best knowledge, this is the first data on evaluation of cements with these specific microbes.

Five cements reported to be used for implant restoration were chosen: zinc oxide eugenol

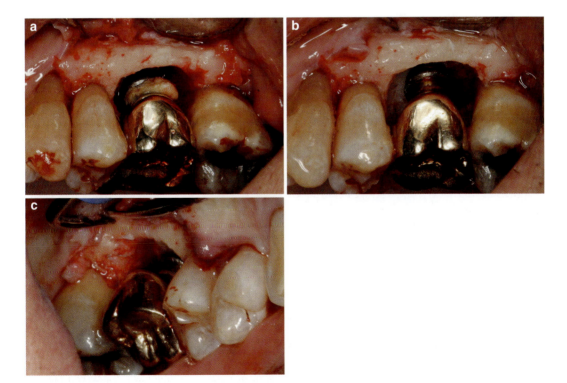

Fig. 3.3 (**a**) Bone loss in a classic crater-type form; excess cement is noted on the implant body. (**b, c**) The crater is noted to extend 360°, with bone loss evident (Photos courtesy of Amy Fuller, DDS, and Brian Fuller, DDS)

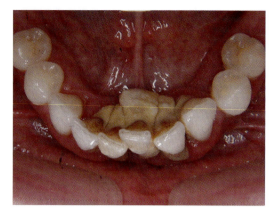

Fig. 3.4 Calculus around these teeth presents an issue due to bacteria associated with it. In itself, it may be considered having more of a "passive" than "active" role in periodontal disease

(TempBond, Kerr), zinc oxide non-eugenol (TempBond NE, Kerr), acrylic urethane (Premier Implant Cement, Premier), zinc orthophosphate (Fleck's, Mizzy); and acrylic (Multilink Implant cement, Ivoclar Vivadent). Disks of the test cement were fabricated under strict aseptic conditions. Bacterial solutions containing individual anaerobic bacterial species were produced. The test cements were placed within the bacterial media and incubated (Fig. 3.9) for 48 hours. Two tests were then done with the cement disks. The first was to determine how they affected the bacteria in the solution (planktonic growth)—were they inhibitors to growth or did the bacteria use the cement as a substrate? The second test compared how many bacteria attached themselves to the cement disk itself (biofilm growth).

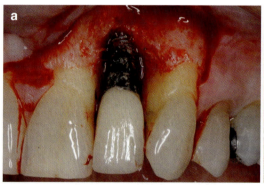
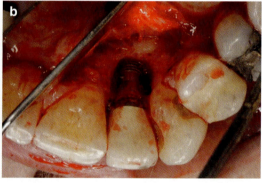

Fig. 3.5 Facial (**a**) and palatal (**b**) photographs of a site affected by residual cement. The resultant disease process is clear. Can this response truly be considered passive like an overhang, or did the cement somehow contribute to the breakdown and have an "active" role?

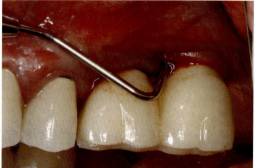
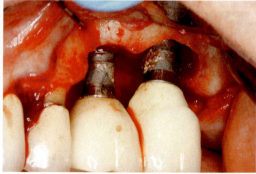

Figs. 3.6 and 3.7 A deep probing noted around these implants. Surgical evaluation with remnants of excess cement noted on these two failing implants. Is it possible so much destruction would have occurred if the cement were simply a passive component in the disease process like an overhang?

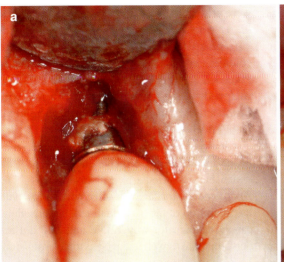
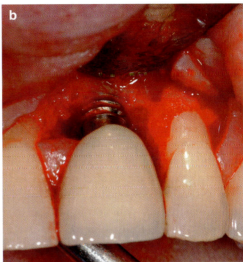

Fig. 3.8 (**a**) Was there always going to be an issue with this implant and the cement is simply there as a result, or did the cement get into the site and cause the problem? (**b**) Debrided site

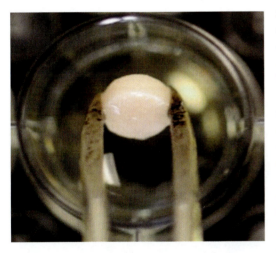

Fig. 3.9 Planktonic growth: test cement disk being introduced into bacteria-containing media

To measure the planktonic effect of the cements, optical density of the solutions was used. In essence, a light beam (wave length 600 nm) was passed through the solution and the opacity measured, which gave an indication of bacterial loading. The opacity of the solution was directly related to the quantity of bacteria present.

The positive control for the planktonic growth was media with bacteria but no cement disk. This represented how the bacteria would grow without external influence. The negative control was the media alone, no bacteria. This was to ensure that none of the samples had any contamination. In effect, the media alone was sterile and appeared clear. The positive and negative controls were used as reference markers against which the cement in bacterial media could be compared (Fig. 3.10a, b).

The results indicated a distinct pattern with respect to planktonic growth, with some cements inhibiting bacterial growth in the media, in some instances reducing the bacterial load to a degree comparative with the negative control. This was most frequently noted with the zinc oxide-containing cements. In contrast, Multilink had very little effect on bacterial inhibition; in some cases it even appeared to promote bacterial growth compared to the positive control (bacteria grown without cement in media), as expressed in Figs. 3.11, 3.12, and 3.13.

Once it was established that differences among the cement samples existed with respect to how they may change the microbial environment into which they are placed, the second study was done. This was to evaluate if there was a difference in adhesion of these Gram-negative bacteria to the cement disk. All the disks were made in a similar manner under aseptic conditions by mixing the cement on sterile pads according to the manufacturer's instructions. The cement was carefully loaded into identical dimension matrix washers then placed between two sterile glass plates and allowed to set. The aim of the glass was to produce similar surface details macroscopically for the test cements. It was understood that the microstructure would differ significantly due to individual cement type differences. The two test cements evaluated were TempBond (having the greatest inhibitory effect on planktonic growth) and Multilink Implant cement (the least inhibitory effect). To determine how many bacteria existed on the cement disks, they were removed from the media after 48 hours incubation, washed in sterile media, and then placed in an Eppendorf Tube with 200 μl of fresh media. The disks were then agitated vigorously to remove the more tightly adherent bacteria. The media was collected and plated on agar plates and incubated under anaerobic conditions.

After 4 days, the colony forming units (CFUs) were recorded for each bacteria–cement combination (Figs. 3.14 and 3.15).

The zinc oxide material (TB) gave, in most instances, no biofilm growth, and where colonies were present, they usually numbered in the order of 12 (some instances with *Porphyromonas gingivalis* [Pg]). By comparison, the number of colonies noted on the ML disks frequently exceeded 5,000 counts; the only exception noted was with some of the plates incubated with *Fusobacterium nucleatum* (Fn), where approximately 150 colonies were counted.

Clearly, this data demonstrates a difference in the interaction of cements and these bacteria which may contribute to a disease process. The zinc cements appeared to offer advantages with the inhibition of the bacteria tested, but this alone cannot account for why TBNE and ZnP did not perform quite as well in the planktonic evaluation.

Zinc has inherent antimicrobial properties. Eugenol is a liquid extract from certain essential oils, especially from clove oil, nutmeg, cinnamon, and bay leaf. Eugenol is well known for its versatile pharmacological actions with anti-inflammatory, anesthetic, antioxidative, and antibacterial properties, even cytotoxic in excess.

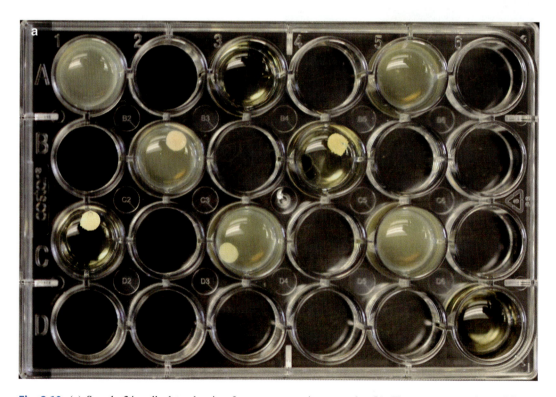

Fig. 3.10 (**a**) Sample 24 well plate showing four test cements and how they affect bacterial planktonic growth. Note the wells that do not contain cement are positive and negative controls. (**b**) These two tests show different results. The opaque test well indicates considerably more growth of bacteria compared to the clearer solution

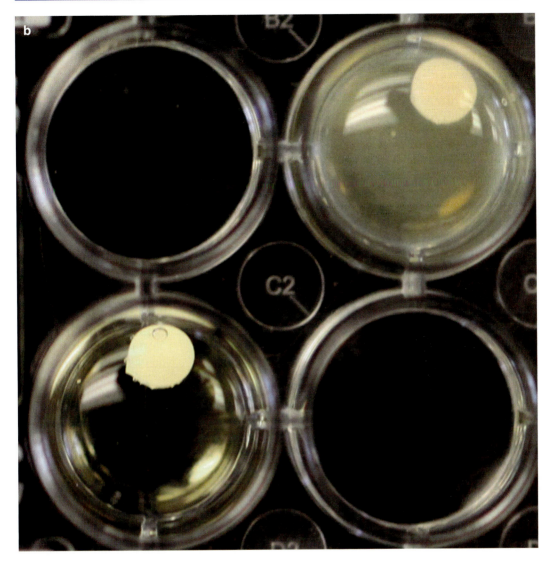

Fig. 3.10 (continued)

Eugenol's cytotoxic properties may be the reason that in this in vitro study the material caused bacterial inhibition. It is believed this to be the first such research paper, and we believe further studies are merited.

The clinical implications related to this study suggest cement selection in specific groups of highly susceptible patients may be based on anti-microbial activity. For example:

1. This is particularly relevant for patients who are periodontally susceptible since this group presents a greater risk to peri-implant disease with the causative microbes frequently being Gram-negative bacteria.

2. Where the implant site is deep within the soft tissues so providing a potentially anaerobic environment.

3. Site known to be infected with these specific bacteria.

Host Response: Foreign Body Reaction

Naomi Ramer has evaluated soft tissue removed from inflammatory sites adjacent to dental implants. Examination has found foreign body reactions; some include giant cell formation. It is

Fig. 3.11 Graph showing mean and standard deviations relating planktonic growth of *Aggregatibacter actinomycetemcomitans* (*Aa*) with the test cements and controls. *TBNE* TempBond NE, *PIC* Premier Implant Cement, *ML* Multilink Implant cement, *ZnP* Fleck's, *TB* TempBond. Positive control—media/bacteria only; Negative control—media only (Reproduced with permission from John Wiley and Sons: Raval et al. (2014). © 2014 Wiley Periodicals, Inc.)

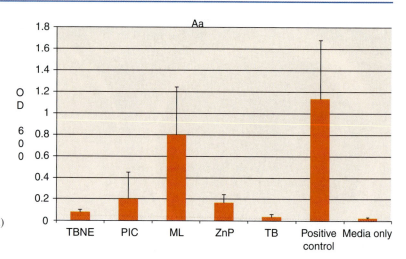

Fig. 3.12 Graph showing mean and standard deviations relating planktonic growth of *Porphyromonas gingivalis* (*Pg*) with the test cements and controls (Reproduced with permission from John Wiley and Sons: Raval et al. (2014). © 2014 Wiley Periodicals, Inc)

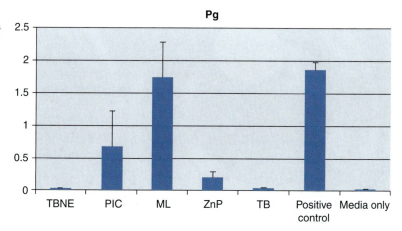

Fig. 3.13 Graph showing mean and standard deviations relating planktonic growth of *Fusobacterium nucleatum* (*Fn*) with the test cements and controls (Reproduced with permission from John Wiley and Sons: Raval et al. (2014). © 2014 Wiley Periodicals, Inc.)

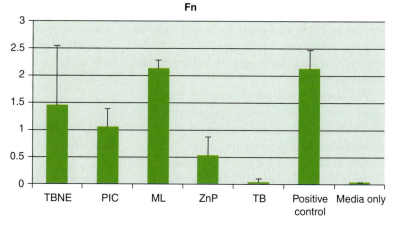

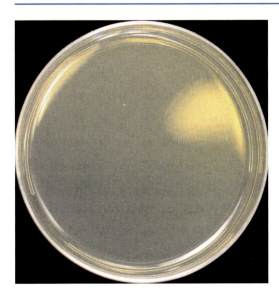

Fig. 3.14 A typical example found with TB with no bio-film growth on the agar plates with *Aggregatibacter actinomycetemcomitans* (Aa) and *Fusobacterium nucleatum* (Fn)

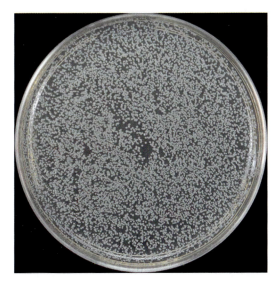

Fig. 3.15 Typical example of biofilm growth found with ML on the agar plates with *Aggregatibacter actinomycetemcomitans* (Aa) and *Porphyromonas gingivalis* (Pg)

possible that in some cases the tissue destruction is host induced as a result of material incorporated within the tissues (Figs. 3.16a, b and 3.17).

One of the components of the human body's cellular defense mechanisms is the macrophage, which is responsible for locating and phagocytosing potentially harmful material. A foreign body

reaction occurs in response to the presence of a foreign entity that is usually too large to be phagocytosed by macrophages (Fig. 3.18). In some instances, the macrophages fuse to form a giant cell. These "super cells" have the ability to secrete degradative agents such as superoxides and free radicals with the goal of destroying the foreign material. However, this is rarely accomplished, and the result is usually mass destruction of the body's own tissues that are adjacent to the site. Some cement remnants have been found within the soft tissues removed from failed implants (Fig. 3.19).

Case Report

A patient presented for routine examination after relocating from another state. She reported no concerns or problems and was seen for routine dental examination. On radiographic examination of the implant site, the prosthodontist noted a crater-type defect associated with the implant around the upper left first molar site (Fig. 3.20a, b).

The patient was informed of the problem and advised to have the site evaluated surgically and debrided. On removal of the crown, the soft tissues appeared somewhat healthy, but deep probing depths were noted (Fig. 3.21a, b).

When the implant was inspected, a "pink"-colored material assumed to be cement was noted on the mesial. It is visible in the photograph (Fig. 3.22a, b). On further investigation, it was discovered that the cement used for this case was Premier Implant Cement—which is pink in color and cannot be detected by radiographic examination further information on cements and radiographic appearance is given in chapter 5. Histopathological reports on the soft tissue harvested at this site describe a foreign body reaction response (Figs. 3.23 and 3.24a, b).

Allergic Response

It has been reported that some of the newer cements contain allergens such as hydroxylated ethylmethacrylate (HEMA). This material has been identified as being extremely irritant to tissues—to the extent that the material safety data sheet states that gloves be worn and the skin and other mucosal tissue such

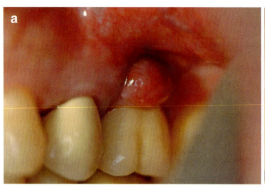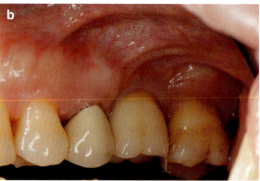

Fig. 3.16 (**a**) Giant cell foreign body reaction associated with residual excess cement. Treatment involved crown removal, lesion excision with debridement, and removal of excess cement. The crown was recemented with greater control and a different cement (TempBond). (**b**) Three-year postoperative view, the lesion has resolved

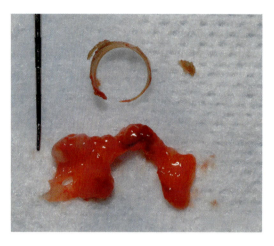

Fig. 3.17 Residual excess cement along with soft tissue. The granulomatous tissue should be sent for histopathologic evaluation

as eyes be protected when used. With subgingival restorative margins frequently employed with cement-retained implant restorations, this is not possible. It is highly possible the cement is leaching out this material prior to setting and producing an immune response (Fig. 3.25a, b).

Alterations in Implant Surfaces

Many cements developed for the natural dentition contain fluoride (to prevent caries when used with a natural tooth restoration). However, it should be noted that fluoride is a chemical known to etch titanium when used in conjunction with an acid. Some cements state clearly in the instructions that they are not suitable for use with titanium structures, yet it appears this is overlooked by many researchers. This omission must be considered a critical error. In 2013, Tarica reported that 17 % of US dental schools selected a polycarboxylate as the final cementing media for implant restorations. Durelon, a popular polycarboxylate, contains fluoride, and a current investigation by the author has shown that this material will corrode titanium. In fact, on the product label, Durelon instructions clearly state that it is not suitable for cementation to titanium.

On further enquiry with 3 M ESPE (e-mail communication by the author), it was determined that the culprit causing corrosion was the stannous fluoride in combination with the polyacrylic acid.

The stannous fluoride was added as a preventative caries agent. This material was specifically designed for natural teeth decades before implant cementation even existed. When this cement is used on implant restorations with the vast majority of implant bodies being composed of titanium alloys, a real risk of an adverse response exists. With 17 % of US dental schools surveyed admitting to its use in 2013, this is a clear indication that instructions are either being ignored or simply not read.

Corrosion is a self-perpetuating physicochemical reaction that results in the reactive oxidative species occurring within the host tissues. This is

Fig. 3.18 A foreign body giant cell reaction. This object is too large for the macrophage to phagocytose. Chemical messages are sent, resulting in collection and fusion of many macrophage cells—the giant cell is formed (Copyright © 2011 Nephron (http://commons.wikimedia. org/wiki/User:Nephron); Permission is granted to copy, distribute, and/or modify this image under the terms of the GNU Free Documentation License Version 1.2 (http:// www.gnu.org/copyleft/fdl. html)) or any later version published by the Free Software Foundation

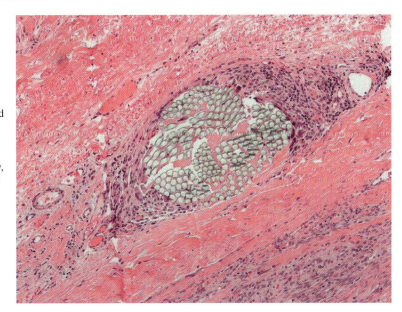

Fig. 3.19 The *dark spots* are cement within this tissue mass of inflammatory tissue. It is possible they contributed to the mass destruction that occurred around this implant

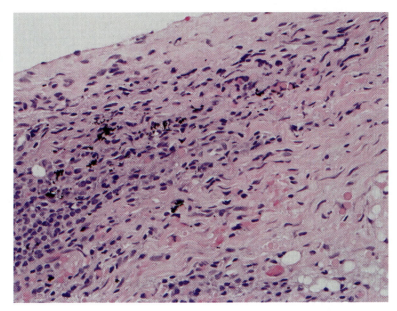

known to cause inflammation and breakdown of the surrounding tissues. Peri-implant disease is such a response. There is no justification for the use of this material where titanium products are used (Fig. 3.26).

Understanding the vulnerabilities of patients is problematic. It is possible that different etiological factors may exist within the same patient or that multiple etiological factors may coexist. If the cementation process is controlled, then all four etiological factors may be eliminated.

Mechanisms of Cement Expression Around a Dental Implant

One question that must be asked is how the cement managed to get within the tissues in the first instance. Understanding the weak soft tissue

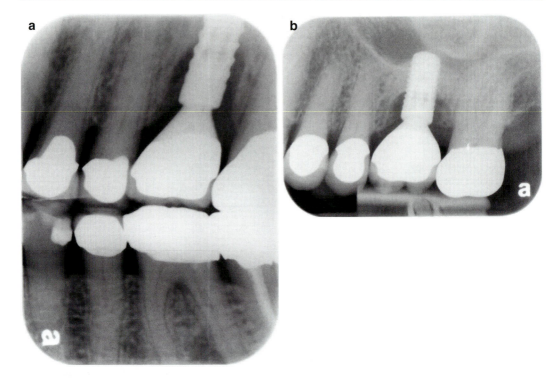

Fig. 3.20 (**a**, **b**) Routine radiographs indicate an issue with this implant. The patient was not experiencing discomfort and was unaware of a problem (Courtesy of Dr. Goichi Shiotsu)

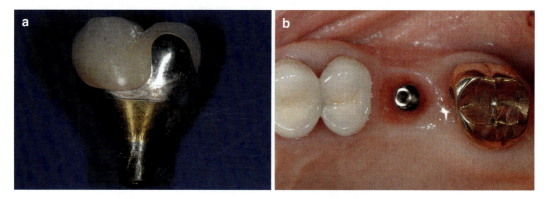

Fig. 3.21 (**a**) The crown and implant abutment were removed by cutting through the occlusal surface to locate the screw. (**b**) The depth of the implant in relation to the size of the crown is shown

attachment coronal to the implant and how it can be easily stripped away with the hydrostatic forces during cement extrusion explains this in part (Fig. 3.27a–c). Linkevičius has also demonstrated that cement is always present on the tissues when cemented margins are placed within the free gingival margins.

One other aspect of the cement getting into the tissues should also be explored. Many of the cement companies have noted that a significant number of crowns fail to seat completely on the abutment. In response, they have developed low-viscosity cement in the belief that this may be advantageous. Some of these cements boast a film thickness of 7 μm. It is seen that whenever a healing cap or other implant component is removed from the implant body, bleeding results. Blood cells have a dimension of

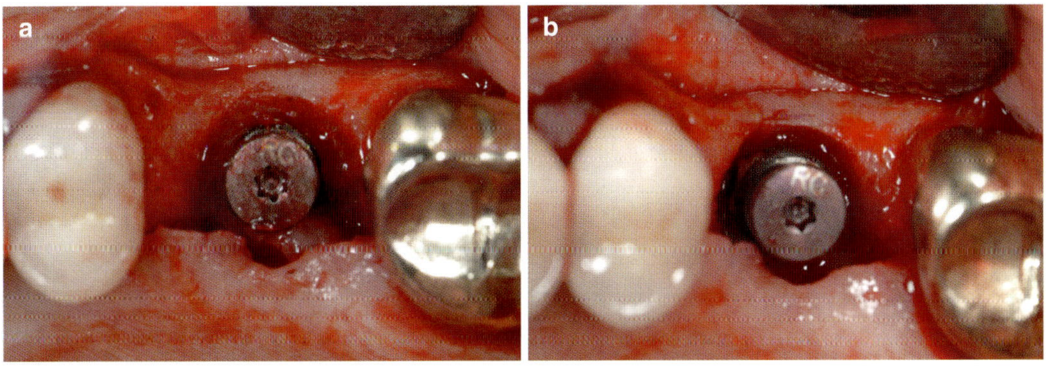

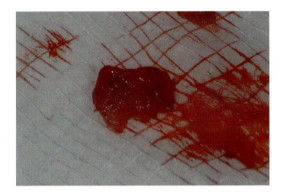

Fig. 3.22 (**a**) Healing cap placed to prevent blood and debris contaminating the internal implant lumen and a full-thickness flap raised. (**b**) On the palatal aspect, a soft tissue mass was noted and removed, pink colored foreign material is seen attached to the mesiall aspect of the implant

Fig. 3.23 The soft tissue mass recovered from around the implant. Note the dark inclusions. This was sent for evaluation and oral pathology report case report courtesy of Dr. Goichi Shiotsu

6–8 μm. Therefore, if these red cells can come out of the tissues, it is no stretch of the imagination that cements this thin can inoculate the tissues when the cement is placed under pressure (Fig. 3.28).

Once the soft tissue site has been either stripped away or penetrated by cement, the next barrier is the bone. One comment that is frequently cited is "if the cement got onto the implant surface, then the implant cannot have been fully integrated." This statement indicates misunderstanding of the bone type into which implants are placed. The name "alveolar" actually describes the bone's character; it is called alveolar bone. This means "cavity or hollow,"

explaining that the bone we place implants into is hollow, with marrow spaces and a highly vascular blood supply. The amount of mineralized tissue touching an implant surface of what is considered a well-integrated implant is only 35–40 %. Therefore, the remaining 60–65 % is un-mineralized and likely to afford little, if any, resistance to the flow of cement under pressure. This is a common finding when post-endodontic treatments are reviewed radiographically. Cement is seen highlighting the marrow spaces (Fig. 3.29).

This radiograph of a root canal filled tooth (Fig. 3.30a) demonstrates the alveolar (small cavities) nature of the bone that implants are placed within. It takes no real stretch of the imagination to understand how cement can flow to extreme depths, even around what is considered a "well-integrated implant." The character of bone can be compared to a loaf of bread—although bread has an outer crust, the structure within is "alveolar" in nature (Fig. 3.30b).

A recent examination of failed and returned implants to Nobel Biocare (Yorba Linda, CA) attested to the depth along the implant surface that some cements had reached (Fig. 3.31) further details are given in chapter 2. Using an X-ray spectrometer, the materials could be readily identified from their chemical composition. This provided a means of evaluating where the cement had extruded.

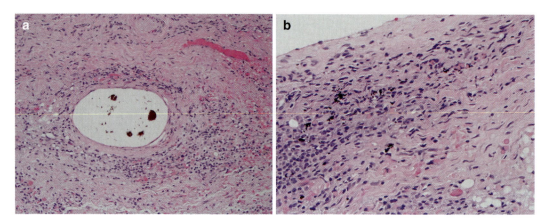

Fig. 3.24 (**a**, **b**) Histological images. The brown-colored material is believed to be cement extrusion products. The pathology report noted "subacutely inflamed granulation tissue, abscess, squamous epithelium, and foreign material"

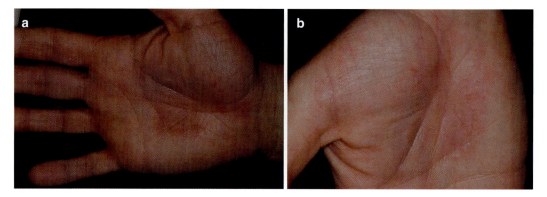

Fig. 3.25 (**a**, **b**) The palm of a dental assistant with contact dermatitis, the result of allergic response to dental materials being handled without barrier protection, i.e., gloves

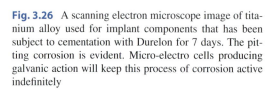

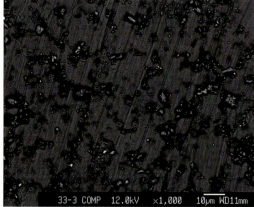

Fig. 3.26 A scanning electron microscope image of titanium alloy used for implant components that has been subject to cementation with Durelon for 7 days. The pitting corrosion is evident. Micro-electro cells producing galvanic action will keep this process of corrosion active indefinitely

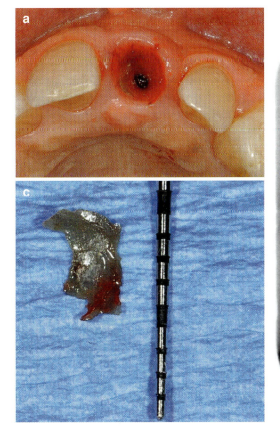

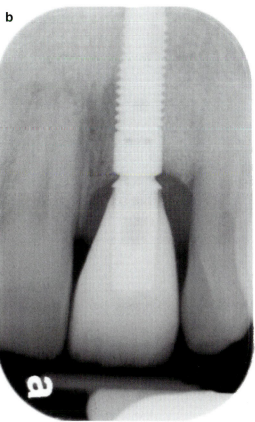

Fig. 3.27 (**a–c**) The hemidesmosomal attachment can be readily detached from the implant by excess cement being forced beyond the margins of the abutment. (**a**) This case demonstrated cement displacement on the soft tissue surfaces when cemented abutment: crown margins are situated below the gingival margin. (**b**) The radiograph did not show cement on the mesial aspect. (**c**) Cement remnants removed, next to a periodontal probe with markings

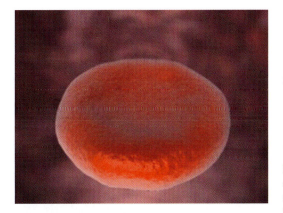

Fig. 3.28 Red blood cell dimension is 6–8 μm. Some cements have film thicknesses of 7 μm

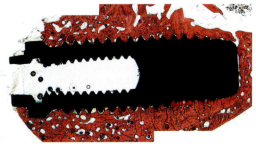

Fig. 3.29 Image of an implant. Although we consider it surrounded by bone, only 35–40 % of the surface is in contact with mineralized tissue. The rest can be in contact with blood vessels, marrow space contents, and fatty tissue. Many of these provide little if any resistance to the flow of cement under pressure reprinted with permission by dentistry Today (Wadhwani 2013b)

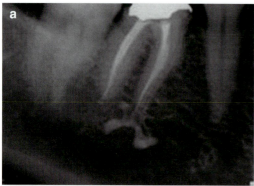

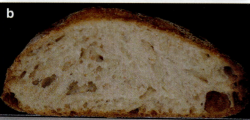

Fig. 3.30 The bone marrow spaces (**a**) This root canal filling material extrusion highlights the bone character and resemble the air spaces seen in common bread (**b**). This provides a good visual to assist in understanding how little resistance there is to the flow of cement (Reprinted with permission by *Dentistry Today* (Wadhwani (2013))

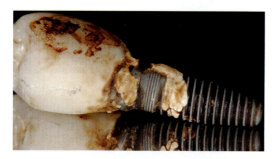

Fig. 3.31 This implant had material one-third along the body length. Evaluation by spectrometer profiling identified this had chemistry consistent with luting cement (see Chap. 2)

Conclusion

The way in which cement may lead to peri-implant diseases is still unknown. A link is apparent and residual excess cement is considered a real issue. The restoring clinician is responsible for how and where cement flows; when it remains within the peri-implant tissues and a disease process results, it must be considered iatrogenic. The cements selected for implant restoration are arbitrarily chosen by the vast majority of clinicians. The main focus for selection appears to be retentive capability, because of familiarity and because they are used for natural teeth. The biological consequences of not fully assessing how the cement will interact with bacteria, the host, or the materials involved are an oversight that could result in peri-implant disease. The clinician must be aware of why implant restorations in particular have vulnerabilities and how to best control them.

Bibliography

Bumgardner JD, Adatrow P, Haggard WO, Norowski PA. Emerging antibacterial biomaterial strategies for the prevention of peri-implant inflammatory diseases. Int J Oral Maxillofac Implants. 2011;26(3):553–60.

Callam D, Cobb C. Excess cement and peri-implant disease. J Implant Adv Clin Dent. 2009;1:61–8.

Coogan MM, Creaven PJ. Antibacterial properties of eight dental cements. Int Endod J. 1993;26:355–61.

Freire MO, Sedghizadeh PP, Schaudinn C, Gorur A, Downey JS, Choi JH, et al. Development of an animal model for Aggregatibacter actinomycetemcomitans biofilm-mediated oral osteolytic infection: a preliminary study. J Periodontol. 2011;82(5):778–89.

Lang NP, Berglundh T, Working Group 4 of Seventh European Workshop on Periodontology. Periimplant diseases: where are we now? – Consensus of the Seventh European Workshop on Periodontology. J Clin Periodontol. 2011;38 Suppl 11:178–81.

Lee A, Wang HL. Biofilm related to dental implants. Implant Dent. 2010;19(5):387–93.

Liddelow G, Klineberg I. Patient-related risk factors for implant therapy. A critique of pertinent literature. Aust Dent J. 2011;56:417–26.

Meffert RM. Periodontitis vs. peri-implantitis: the same disease? The same treatment? Crit Rev Oral Biol Med. 1996;7(3):278–91. 3.

Mombelli A, Décaillet F. The characteristics of biofilms in peri-implant disease. J Clin Periodontol. 2011;38 Suppl 11:203–13.

Pjetursson BE, Helbling C, Weber HP, Matuliene G, Salvi GE, Brägger U, et al. Peri-implantitis susceptibility as it relates to periodontal therapy and supportive care. Clin Oral Implants Res. 2012;23(7):888–94.

Pramod K, Ansari SH, Ali J. Eugenol: a natural compound with versatile pharmacological actions. Nat Prod Commun. 2010;5(12):1999–2006.

Ramer N, Wadhwani C, Kim A, Hershman D. Histologic findings within peri-implant soft tissue in failed implants secondary to excess cement: report of two cases and review of literature. NY State Dent J. 2014;80:43–6.

Rosen P, Clem D, Cochran D, Froum S, et al. Academy report: Peri-Implant Mucositis and Peri-Implantitis. A current understanding of their diagnoses and clinical implications. J periodontol. 2013;84:436–43.

Raval NC, Wadhwani CPK, Jain S, Darveau RP. The interaction of implant luting cements and oral bacteria linked to peri-implant disease; an in-vitro analysis of planktonic and biofilm growth – a preliminary study. Clin Implant Dent Relat Res. 2014 Jun 6. doi: 10.1111/cid.12235. [Epub ahead of print].

Rosenstiel SF, Land MF, Crispin BJ. Dental luting agents: a review of the current literature. J Prosthet Dent. 1998;80(3):280–301.

Tarica DY, Alvarado VM, Truong ST. Survey of United States dental schools on cementation protocols for implant crown restorations. J Prosthet Dent. 2010;103:68–79.

Wadhwani CPK. Peri-implant disease and cemented implant restorations: a multifactorial etiology. Compend Contin Educ Dent. 2013a;34 Spec No 7:32–7.

Wadhwani CP, Schwedhelm ER. The role of cements in dental implant success, part 1. Dent Today. 2013;32(4):76.

Wadhwani CP, Pineyro AF. Implant cementation: clinical problems and solutions. Dent Today. 2012;31(1):56. 58, 60–2.

Wilson TG. The positive relationship between excess cement and peri-implant disease: a prospective clinical endoscopic study. J Periodontol. 2009;80:1388–92.

Implant Luting Cements

4

Chandur P.K. Wadhwani,
Ernesto Ricardo Schwedhelm,
Diane Yoshinobu Tarica,
and Kwok-Hung (Albert) Chung

Abstract

Dental luting cements have in general been exclusively designed for the natural tooth, with features that allow for reduction in caries, adhesion to natural tooth tissues, and radiographic appearance often related to dentine. Although many of these properties are redundant when considering restoring dental implants, studies show clinicians frequently do not take this into account. This chapter deals with ideal cement selection criteria and compares this to what is actually being used in teaching institutions. Cementation procedures are poorly understood especially site and amount application which greatly affect cement extrusion. The second part relates more specifically to modeling cement flow and how understanding the non-Newtonian properties of cements is vital to implant success. Computational fluid dynamic studies similar to those used in all forms of engineering will become the gold standard for investigating the cement-retained crown system. Such an approach unites the properties of the crown, the abutment shape, and the cement characteristics into a single functional system, where cement behavior is governed by physical forces. The design of implant components should not be arbitrarily related to tooth preparations; these medical devices should have a design or form that follows function.

C.P.K. Wadhwani, BDS (Hons), MSD (✉)
Department of Restorative Dentistry, University of
Washington School of Dentistry, 1200 116th Ave,
Seattle, WA 98004, USA

University of Washington School of Dentistry,
Seattle, WA, USA
e-mail: cpkw@uw.edu

E.R. Schwedhelm, DDS, MSD, FRCDC
Department of Restorative Dentistry, University of
Washington, School of Dentistry, Seattle, WA, USA

Private Practice Limited to Prosthodontics,
Seattle, WA, USA

D.Y. Tarica, DDS, FACP
Private Practice Limited to Prosthodontics,
Los Angeles, CA, USA

K-H. Chung, DDS, PhD
Department of Restorative Dentistry, University of
Washington School of Dentistry, Seattle, WA, USA

C.P.K. Wadhwani (ed.), *Cementation in Dental Implantology: An Evidence-Based Guide*,
DOI 10.1007/978-3-642-55163-5_4, © Springer-Verlag Berlin Heidelberg 2015

Cement Selection for Implant Restoration

Since the introduction of single and multiple implant prosthesis, cement- and screw-retained implant restorations are accepted treatment options for the replacement of missing teeth (Fig. 4.1a–d). Over the years, dental implants have achieved a high success rate and are considered the standard care for the replacement of missing teeth.

With the continuous success of dental implant restorations, constant innovations have been presented to the dental profession to improve the position of implants, esthetics, and control of occlusion to facilitate ideal restorative procedures.

Initially, implant prostheses were almost entirely screw retained until the early 1990s, when two of the foremost implant manufacturers, Straumann and Nobel Biocare, developed cementable abutment options. Today, implant manufacturers offer several options for screw- and cement-retained restorations. The screw-retained prostheses have the advantage of retrievability over cement-retained restorations; however, screw loosening was an initial issue encountered by many implant restoring clinicians. It is widely

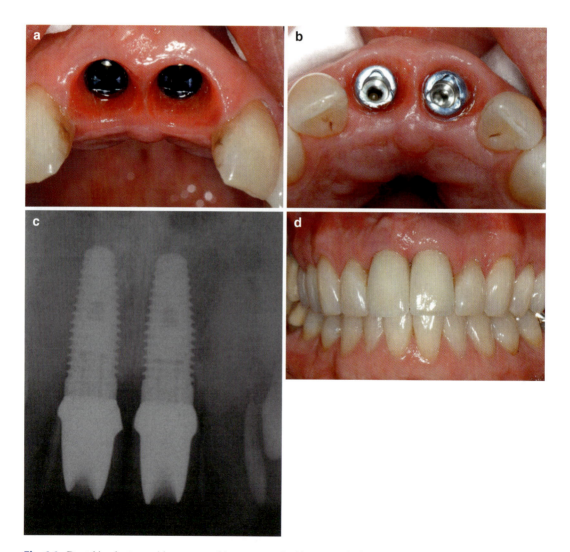

Fig. 4.1 Dental implants provide an acceptable treatment, in this case replacing the central incisors. (**a**) The soft tissue emergence profile of the implants. (**b**) Occlusal view. (**c**) Radiograph of the final restorations. (**d**) Completed Restorations

thought that this was mainly due to the inadequate tightening of the screw. Torque wrenches were not widely used during restorative procedures, resulting in little, if any, preload being applied to the screw. With no clamping forces, the screw joint would be destined to fail under cyclic loading in the oral environment.

Studies have shown that screw loosening is, in fact, a rare event. Theoharidou et al. published a systematic review on abutment screw loosening in single implant restorations. Their conclusions were that abutment screw loosening occurred as a rare event, regardless of the connection geometry of the implant to abutment, provided proper anti-rotational features and torque were employed. The early failures due to screw loosening led to the use of provisional cements to assist in maintaining the retrievability of cemented prostheses. However, with the current success and predictability of implant restorations, manufacturers are recommending a wide variety of cements, from provisional to definitive resin-based cements. Several authors have suggested that the advantages of cement-retained implant restorations include the following: more passive fit of the casting, improved direction of the load, enhanced esthetics, improved access, progressive loading, and reduced crestal bone loss. Some disadvantages include low profile retention, limited interarch space, retrievability, and presence of cement in sulcus. However, it is more likely that cement-retained restorations have been a restorative treatment of choice by the dental profession due to the familiarized routine of the fabrication of cement-retained tooth restorations. These techniques are well established and were thought to be well understood.

Material Selection: Teeth Versus Implants

Dental cements have been manufactured for use with the natural dentition. The authors have not found any cement that was solely developed for the implant restoration. As a result, the properties of cements are designed to have an interaction with the natural tooth. For example, many release fluoride as an anticaries agent, some cements etch

dentine, some chelate to the calcium ion found in tooth tissue, etc. None of these properties are required with dental implants. In fact, some are detrimental with certain implant materials.

Currently there is no ideal cement manufactured for the cementation of implant-supported restorations. The list of available cements is diverse, and it is important that the dental practitioner fully understands that there are different requirements between a natural tooth and the dental implant abutment.

Wadhwani and Schwedhelm summarized in detail the different considerations for material selection specific to teeth and implant-cemented restorations (Table 4.1).

There is no consensus on which cement or material is the most appropriate for cementing implant restorations. Tarica has recorded information on US dental schools and their teaching recommendations for implant restorations.

Table 4.1 Some of the differences in cement selection criteria for implant restorations and cement properties for the natural tooth

	Implant restoration	Natural tooth
Substructure	Metal, ceramic, acrylic	Dentine, enamel
Biological tissue association	Peri-implant tissues	Periodontal tissues, pulp
Primary disease issue	Peri-implant disease	Caries, pulpal, periodontal
Restorations finish line	1–2 mm below the gingiva crest, frequently deeper	1/2–1 mm below anterior esthetic sites, often above free gingival margins
Cement margin	May or may not follow scallop of tissues	Preparation follow gingival tissues
Need for cement seal	Questionable	Absolute (prevent caries)
Anticaries agents	May be detrimental	Desirable
Corrosion	Corrosion of titanium possible	Not applicable
Radiopacity	Highly radiopaque	Similar to dentine (relatively low)
Microbial challenge	Bacteria found in peri-implant sites	Caries-producing bacteria

Survey of US Dental Schools

Two separate surveys in 2008 and 2013 were sent to US dental schools on cementation protocols for implant crown restorations. Although a wide variety of cementation preparations and materials were reported, the surveys revealed some commonly used implant techniques taught at US dental schools. A total of 69 surveys were returned in 2013, representing 65 dental schools and 42 prosthodontic programs. After deleting duplicate responses, 42 surveys were returned from restorative departmental chairpersons, and 27 from advanced prosthodontic residency directors. The new dental schools reported that they did not have a protocol in place yet.

Cement Selection

Some changes were noted in the cement selection between 2008 (Fig. 4.2) and 2013 (Fig. 4.3). Although most institutions taught the use of definitive cement for inserting the final implant prosthesis, there are no standards for cement selection for implant restorations, even within the same institution.

A resin-modified glass ionomer cement was found to be the most commonly used among both restorative departments (57 %) and advanced prosthodontic programs (59 %). Advanced prosthodontic programs included glass ionomer (19 %), resin cement (52 %), zinc phosphate (33 %), and polycarboxylate (22 %) cements. The restorative departments taught the use of the following definitive cements: glass ionomer (19 %), resin (33 %), zinc phosphate (19 %), and polycarboxylate cement (17 %).

Provisional cements, ZOE based, were widely used by predoctoral (40 %) and postgraduate (33 %) programs. Some institutions explained that they used a provisional cement to maintain retrievability or to ensure that the restoration was satisfactory prior to using a more retentive cement. The survey also asked the respondents what cements were used for conventional fixed restorations. Eighty-seven percent of the restorative departments taught the use of resin-modified glass ionomer, followed by composite resin, glass ionomer, and zinc phosphate. Acrylic urethane cements were also taught by 14 % of the predoctoral programs. Seventy percent of advanced prosthodontic directors taught the use

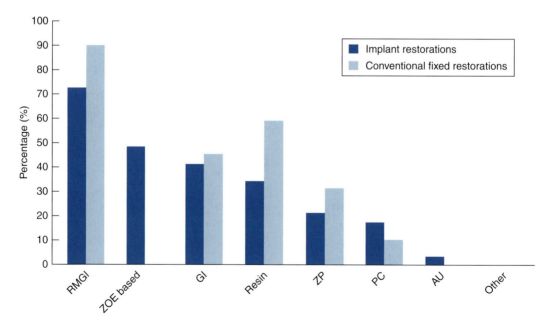

Fig. 4.2 Definitive cements used for implant and conventional fixed restorations by prosthodontic residency directors in 2008. *RMGI* resin-modified glass ionomer, *ZOE* zinc oxide eugenol, *GI* glass ionomer, *ZP* zinc phosphate, *PC* polycarboxylate, *AU* acrylic urethane (Reprinted from the Tarica et al. (2010). Copyright © 2010, with permission from Elsevier)

Fig. 4.3 Definitive cements used for implant and conventional fixed restorations by prosthodontic residency directors in 2013. *RMGI* resin-modified glass ionomer, *ZOE* zinc oxide eugenol, *GI* glass ionomer, *ZP* zinc phosphate, *PC* polycarboxylate, *AU* acrylic urethane

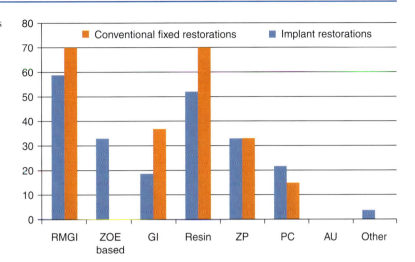

of resin-modified glass ionomer and resin, glass ionomer, zinc phosphate, and polycarboxylate cements. Both predoctoral and postgraduate programs showed an increase in the use of resin cements and slight decrease of use of resin-modified glass ionomer cements between the 2008 and 2013 surveys, for both implant and conventional fixed restorations. With the increased availability of various all-ceramic restorations, this may have led to the increased use of resin cements for conventional fixed restorations and correspondingly to implant restorations. In general, there seems to be a similarity with cements used for implant restorations, which indicates that the same cements were probably selected from convenience, familiarity, and cost. Some of the literature has shown that the retentiveness of a particular cement for natural dentition may not correlate with implant components. Therefore, until more data is available, the clinician may or may not have the expected retention from the same cement for implant restorations.

The last question on the survey asked if there were any changes in cement for specific clinical situations. Of the 20 predoctoral and postgraduate programs that completed this section, the only trend seen was that a resin cement was used for either a zirconium- or aluminum-based abutment. A few responded that they changed cements depending on the type of ceramic used for the restoration. With regard to abutment and/or restorative material and design, the responses were few and, again, ranged from provisional to definitive cements. Since most of the schools did not respond to this question and there was great variability in cement types, it was assumed that, in general, the same cement is used for most all clinical situations.

Implant System Selection

Implants from various implant manufacturers are used at US dental institutions (Fig. 4.4). The 2013 survey showed the implant manufacturers most used, in order, were as follows: Nobel Biocare, Straumann, Biomet 3i, Astra Tech, and Zimmer. Other implant manufacturers were generally used by less than 37 % of dental schools; however, from 2008 to 2013, this group had increased from 21 %.

Although some schools used up to nine different implant manufacturer systems, most dental schools used only between one to four varieties. Differences also existed among departments in the same school as to the preference of implants used.

Abutment Selection

Schools were asked for their preference to abutment selection. Restorative chairpersons and prosthodontic residency directors responded that they mostly used either prefabricated abutments or the computer-aided, custom-milled abutments. Since the recent expense in gold and the introduction of computer-milled, custom abutments, the survey indicates that traditional custom cast, UCLA-type abutments, are used infrequently.

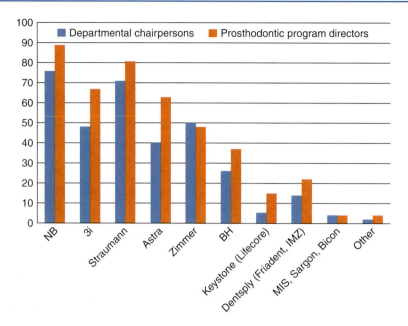

Fig. 4.4 Implant manufacturers used at US dental institutions in 2013. *NB* Nobel Biocare AB (Gothenburg, Sweden), *3i* Biomet 3i Inc (Palm Beach Gardens), *Straumann* Institut Straumann AG (Basel, Switzerland), *Astra* Astra Tech Inc (Waltham, MA), *Zimmer* Zimmer Dental (Carlsbad, CA), *BH* BioHorizons (Birmingham, AL), *Keystone* Dentsply (Mannheim, Germany), *MIS* MIS Implants Technologies Ltd (Shlomi, Israel), *Sargon* Sargon Dental Implants (Encino, CA), *Bicon* Bicon (Boston, MA), *Other* OsseoLink, Global Implant Solutions LLC (Bedford, MA), and Hiossen Inc (Fairless Hills, PA) (Used with permission from Wadhwani et al. (2012). Copyright © Quintessence Publishing Company, Inc., Chicago, IL USA)

Abutment Modifications

The survey also included the different surface preparations to either the implant abutment or the restoration prior to final cementation. Most institutions kept the preparation simple with either no modification or only one modification prior to inserting the definitive implant prosthesis. The most common procedure for both predoctoral and postgraduate programs was application of airborne-particle abrasion aluminum oxide to the internal surface of the implant restoration prior to cementation (Fig. 4.5).

The department chairpersons also indicated that students applied a ceramic primer to the intaglio of the restoration (35 %). Thirty-three percent indicated that grooves were added to the implant abutment to increase the resistance to retention and total convergence angle for the definitive implant cement-retained restorations. Other procedures taught by less than 14 % of predoctoral programs were polishing or abrading the implant abutment with a rotary instrument and the application of a metal primer, tin-plating, or placing a vent hole. Fifty-two percent of the prosthodontic residency directors applied a ceramic primer to

ceramic restorations (Table 4.2). In a 2008 survey, only 3 % had reported placing a primer to ceramic restorations. This may indicate an increased use and confidence in cementing all-ceramic restorations on zirconium abutments. Nineteen percent of prosthodontic residency directors reported the placement of grooves on the implant abutments, as well as airborne-particle abrasion of the implant abutment. They also indicated that they polished the abutment, abraded the abutments with a rotary instrument, or used tin-plating to prepare the abutment or restoration prior to cementation. None of the postgraduate programs placed vent holes to aid in cementation. Some schools commented that they prepared the abutment and restoration the same way as cementing to natural dentition.

Immediate Provisionalization

This was taught to predoctoral students in about 55 % of the dental schools and 70 % of the postdoctoral prosthodontic programs. For both pre- and postdoctoral programs, the preferred design for immediate provisionalization was screw-retained restorations. For the few that cemented their

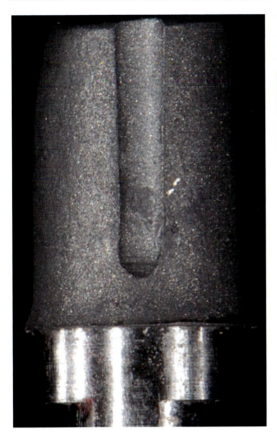

Fig. 4.5 An example of abutment modifications. This abutment has been air abraded and also has an axial groove placed. This would represent two modifications

Table 4.2 Frequency (%) of preparations for implant abutment and/or restoration prior to definitive cementation by department chairpersons ($n=42$) and prosthodontic residency directors ($n=27$)

Abutment modifications 2013	Departmental chairpersons	Prosthodontic residency directors
Airborne-particle abrasion of internal surface of restoration	25 (60 %)	15 (56 %)
No modifications or preparations	7 (17 %)	2 (7 %)
Grooves placed on abutment	14 (33 %)	5 (19 %)
Airborne-particle abrasion of abutment	6 (14 %)	7 (26 %)
Polishing abutment	2 (5 %)	4 (15 %)
Application of metal or ceramic primer	15 (35 %)	14 (52 %)
Abrading abutment with rotary instrument	0	1 (4 %)
Tin-plating	0	1 (4 %)
Placement of vent hole	1 (2 %)	0
Other	0	0

provisional restorations, many schools noted that a temporary abutment was placed and the restoration was temporarily cemented.

Management of the Screw Access Channel

Both predoctoral and postdoctoral programs used various types and number of materials to fill the screw access hole. However, most taught their students and residents to fill the screw access completely to the top of the abutment. In 2008, 71 and 86 % of restorative and prosthodontic programs indicated that they teach their students/residents to fill the screw access opening completely. In 2013, the numbers declined slightly to 69 and 67 %, respectively. The survey did not ask for a specific reason; however, more schools may be concerned about controlling the flow of material during cementation. Several different materials and combinations of materials were used to fill the abutment screw access hole. Most schools seemed to use two to three materials, with a range of one to five for predoctoral and one to eight different materials for prosthodontic directors. The major difference between the surveys conducted in 2008 and 2013 was the increased use in PTFE tape as a material to fill the screw access. Table 4.3 shows the most frequently used combination of materials in 2008—note that PTFE (Polytetrafluoroethylene tape or plumbers tape) did not appear on this list. Both restorative and departmental chairpersons and prosthodontic residency directors most frequently filled the screw access hole with a cotton pellet followed by composite, or PTFE tape followed by composite.

Summary

No ideal cement exists, but what is apparent is that little, if any, thought is provided to the choice of material used. Within the dental schools, it appears arbitrary, with the choice for implant restoration commonly reflecting the choice for cementation of crowns and bridges on natural teeth. This oversight is problematic, especially as some cements are detrimental to the materials used in implant. There appears to be little consensus on the most appropriate abutment management also, with differences in

Table 4.3 Frequency (%) of usage of various materials for filling screw access opening

Material	Departmental chairpersons 2008	Departmental chairpersons 2013	Prosthodontic residency directors 2008	Prosthodontic residency directors 2013
Cotton Pellet	24 (77 %)	28 (67 %)	17 (59 %)	16 (59 %)
PTFE	0	20 (48 %)	0	14 (52 %)
Gutta-percha	12 (39 %)	5 (12 %)	9 (31 %)	6 (22 %)
Light-cured temp.	12 (39 %)	9 (21 %)	8 (28 %)	17 (63 %)
Composite	16 (52 %)	17 (40 %)	18 (62 %)	22 (81 %)
Acrylic	0	1 (2 %)	0	3 (11 %)
Rubber material	13 (42 %)	15 (36 %)	12 (41 %)	17 (63 %)
Amalgam	1 (3 %)	0	1 (3 %)	4 (15 %)
Glass ionomer	1 (3 %)	1 (2 %)	1 (3 %)	0
Cavit	7 (23 %)	10 (24 %)	1 (3 %)	3 (11 %)
IRM	1 (3 %)	2 (5 %)	0	0
Other	1 (3 %)	1 (2 %)	4 (14 %)	3 (11 %)

different departments even within the same institution. There is a clear need to develop protocols more closely related to scientific enquiry than anecdotal processes.

Understanding and Controlling Cement Flow

Cementation as a means of attaching a restoration—such as an inlay, onlay, crown, or bridge—to a natural tooth has been used for close to 100 years. The process serves to unite components of the same or different materials together. The cementing media used can result in a union that is primarily frictional (e.g., zinc phosphate cement), where some form of mechanical or micro-mechanical interlocking occurs, adhesive in nature where a chemical bond unites the structures (e.g., self-etching resin systems and dentine), or both, depending on the materials joined.

With the advent of dental implants and the subsequent introduction of the cement-retained implant restoration came the emergence of new issues that are not commonly seen to occur when restoring teeth. The cement-retained implant restoration may be more vulnerable to the effects of cement flowing into the soft tissues and residual excess cement on the implant restoration when compared to a tooth. Although there are tens of thousands of articles written on cements, highlighting tensile, shear strengths, their properties, and clinical applications, very little is reported about the way in which cements flow during

the cementation process, how to optimize their application, or the amount of cement required to achieve the ideal cementation results.

The occlusion of the cemented crown can be altered by the quality and quantity of cement applied to the internal aspect of the crown. This has been reported by several who have studied cement application techniques with respect to vertical displacement.

Having a sealed restorative margin is considered a prerequisite for a tooth to eliminate ingress of bacteria that could cause subsequent caries. With implant restorations, a bacterial marginal seal provided by cement lute may not be a great concern, especially when one considers the success that screw-retained restorations have, where no seal exists. Marginal adaptation of an implant crown has not been shown to be problematic; Jemt found no issue with the exposed set cement that filled the marginal space between the implant abutment and crown. Marginal seal may, however, be important with respect to cement lute washout during (contamination from crevicular fluids) and after luting (dissolution of the cement) the restoration. Residual excess cement extrusion from around the margin of the cemented restoration of implants is a problem that has also been described in the literature.

Survey: How Much Cement Should We Use?

A recent survey of more than 400 dentists evaluated cement application techniques specifically

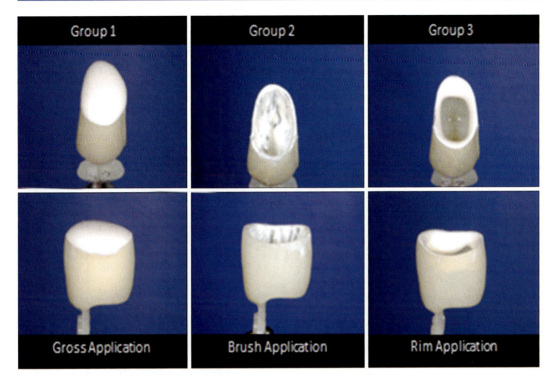

Fig. 4.6 Actual examples of loading patterns and site of cement from a survey of more than 400 dentists on how they place cement for an implant crown (Used with permission from Wadhwani et al. (2012). Copyright © Quintessence Publishing Company, Inc., Chicago, IL USA)

for implant crowns. The data revealed a large difference in application technique and site. Most dentists (55 %) applied cement on the internal surface with a brush, 28 % of those surveyed applied cement arbitrarily by loading the inside of the crown, and a smaller proportion (17 %) preferentially loaded the internal margin of the crown (Fig. 4.6). From this study, there appeared to be little consensus on the most appropriate site or technique when considering cementation of implant crowns.

A second part of the survey involved weighing the amount of cement placed into the crowns and comparing it to the ideal amount required such that the crown completely seated, with complete cement lute space filled with cement and no excess. This was determined to be 3 % of the total crown volume. What was of significant interest was the range of cement placed within the crowns. Some surveyed dentists loaded the crowns with greater than 50 times the amount of cement required. Others placed only one-quarter of the ideal amount needed (Fig. 4.7a, b).

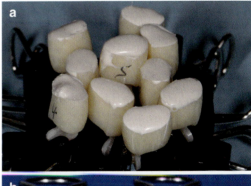

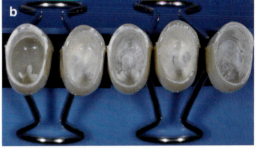

Fig. 4.7 (a) This group of dentists overfilled the crowns with cement—some placed over 50 times the ideal amount required. (b) This group underfilled the crowns with insufficient cement to fill the lute space

Fig. 4.8 A box-and-whisker graph indicating how the choice of cement application site relates to the amount of cement used

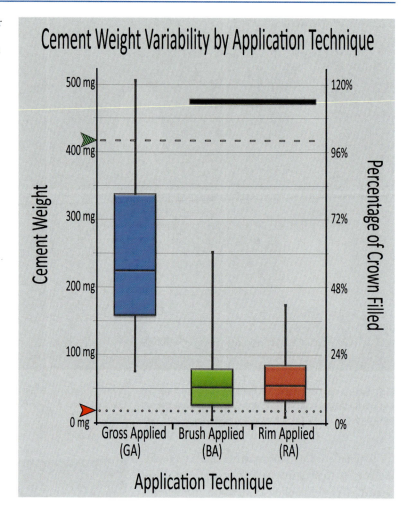

The clinical significance of the cement application and volume data indicates a large variation in thought processes, with very few dentists able to provide the appropriate volume of cement (Fig. 4.8). Too little cement and the crown may not stay on; too much cement may result in cement extrusion into the tissues and result in peri-implant disease.

It should be understood that the laboratories fabricating the restorations provide the clinician with a limited finite volume for cement in some form of relief, usually a die spacer, either painted onto the abutment, if fabricated by conventional dental techniques, or "built-in" with CAD/CAM technology. This usually equates to about 20–50 µm of space or as thick as a one to two layers of nail varnish!

Cements as Fluids

Clinicians should be aware of how materials such as fluids behave. While this is beyond the scope of this text, a very brief summary will be given. Cements vary in their physical nature, predominantly dependent upon their chemical composition, but in general, cements are considered viscous fluids. Fluids can be loosely defined by their behavior when exposed to an applied force. Most common liquids for example, water is Newtonian in nature, which means when a force is applied, the viscosity remains unchanged. In essence, they flow and take up the shape of the container that houses them (Fig. 4.9a).

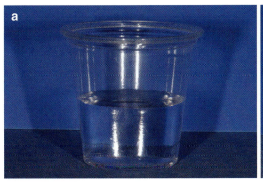

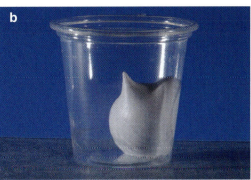

Fig. 4.9 (**a**) This body of water has Newtonian proper-ties; it fills this container and will flow according to Newtonian laws when a force is applied to it. (**b**) This liquid does not follow Newtonian laws. It does not flow into the container and will behave differently than water when force is applied

In dentistry, most polymers (many cements are polymers) are considered non-Newtonian liquids. Although they may appear as liquids, they have unusual flow properties. These materials are not displaced by forces and do not flow into containers like water does (Fig. 4.9b). This can be of advan-tage; consider placing a cement within a crown and inverting it. If it had water-like properties, it would flow out immediately; with non-Newtonian properties, it would remain where it was placed.

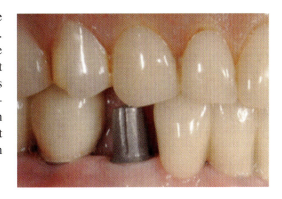

Fig. 4.10 Typical form of a posterior implant abutment: Flattop cone, circular in cross section, and occlusal con-vergence taper 6–10°

Modeling Cement Flow: A Simple Demonstration

The implant abutment onto which a restoration is subsequently cemented generally has a very simple form, usually circular in cross section and similar to a flat-top cone with an occlu-sal convergence taper of approximately 6–10° (Fig. 4.10).

Cement flow can be easily modeled to dem-onstrate the influence of the following variables: placement site, amount used, and abutment mod-ifications. To do this, the model system should allow the cement flow to be visualized. In other words, the model system should ideally be trans-parent. The two-model structures should conform to the shape of a crown and the implant abutment.

One simple yet crude model system is to use clear plastic drinking beakers. For demonstration, the flow behavior of cement can be mimicked by using shaving cream (Fig. 4.11a–c).

One documented method for loading cement into a crown prior to seating onto an implant abutment is to arbitrarily or gross-fill the res-toration and then seat it onto the abutment. The amount loaded is usually far in excess of what is required to ideally fill the cement space provided for the clinician during crown fabrication. Often, the crown is further seated by the application of a seating force (the patient bites on a wood stick or cotton wool, holding the restoration as the cement set commences) of around 5 kg. To simulate the cement flow when this technique is used, the crown component of the model sys-tem is half-filled with the shaving foam and then seated onto the beaker representing the implant abutment. The "crown" has to be forced down to overcome the hydrostatic pressure resistance

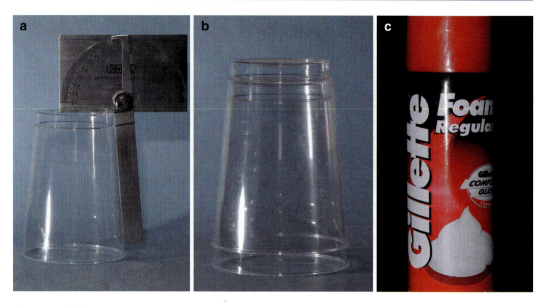

Fig. 4.11 (**a**) The model system: Clear drinking beakers; note total occlusal convergence recorded with a protractor (10° total). (**b**) Beakers are designed to "fit" directly onto one another, similar to a crown and an abutment. (**c**) Shaving foam represents the cement

Fig. 4.12 (**a**) Cement applied in the form of gross application; (**b**) fully seated with excess

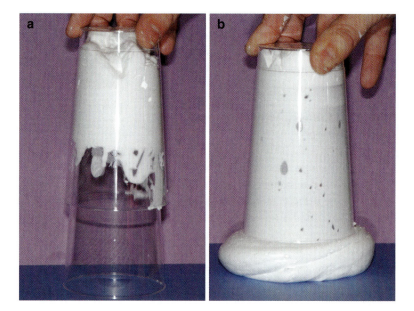

from the occlusal cement layer that traps between the two horizontal surfaces. Liquids (cements prior to setting) are resistant to compression, unlike gases. Once the applied force is great enough to overcome this compression, the cement flows down onto the axial walls of the "abutment" and the excess cement will eventually be extruded out of the crown/abutment margin under great pressure (Fig. 4.12a, b). The pressure may be so great that the vulnerable soft tissue hemidesmosomal attachment to the implant may be damaged and even detached, which could allow cement to flow well beneath the tissues.

Two effects are noted: (1) the occlusal cement is in compression and resists seating

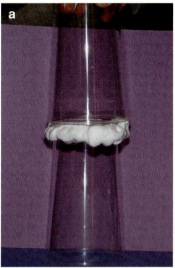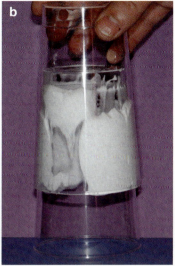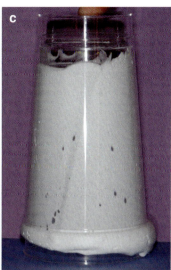

Fig. 4.13 (a–c) Application of cement to the axial wall near but not on the occlusal surface results in the cement flowing in the same direction as the applied seating force. The occlusal aspect remains unfilled and considerably less excess extrusion is noted when compared to the gross application in Fig. 4.12a, b

forces, propping the "crown" up, and (2) the cement extruded is under great force, which may damage the soft tissue attaching to the implant surface. The crown is, on average, 50 % filled with cement, whereas only about 3 % is actually required. Too much is used and most of it must be extruded out of the system. Note the excess and the blanching of the fingers in Fig. 4.12b indicating the amount of force required to seat the "crown." Large amounts of excess cement extruded out through the margin of the crown/abutment because the amount of cement loaded into the crown is poorly controlled.

Some studies have suggested that the axial wall of the abutment near to, but not including, the occlusal surface itself has cement applied to it (Fig. 4.13a–c). When the crown is seated by application of a force the cement is acted upon by shear forces. The result is the cement is forced down the abutment axial walls, leaving a void near the occlusal aspect of the abutment (7). Less excess cement extrusion is seen at the margin when compared to the gross application technique due to less cement material applied in the first instance. However, the incomplete fill of the cement space makes this process potentially problematic with potential reduction of retentive force capabilities.

When the cement is applied to the internal aspect of the crown near to, but not including, the crown margin and then seated onto the abutment, a different effect is seen (Fig. 4.14a–c). The cement appears to flow against the direction of the seating force. In effect, it flows upward. The cement, as the crown is seated, contacts the axial walls of the abutment. The seating force acts to compress the cement against the axial walls, which are round and tapered. This compression forces the cement to flow up, until the occlusal table is reached. At this point, the vector of force no longer acts, as it lies perpendicular to the seating force. The remainder of the cement gets forced down toward the margins, with much less extrusion out than compared with either of the two former techniques. The cement fill is also more ideal.

The cement flow toward the occlusal surface (Fig. 4.15) is of interest especially where implant restorations are involved. It is considered common practice to close off an abutment screw access before the crown is cemented; in fact, all of the US dental schools advocate this (Fig. 4.16).

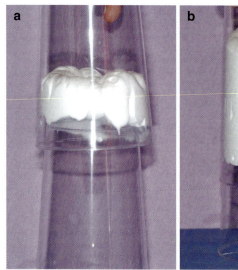
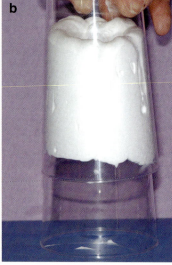
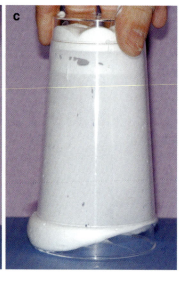

Fig. 4.14 (**a–c**) Application of the cement near to the inner crown margin results in a flow pattern that forces cement occlusally initially, then as the model crown seats, the cement then flows down toward the margin, with small amounts of excess cement

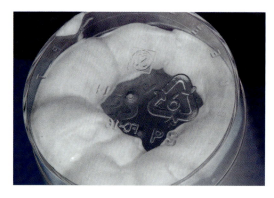

Fig. 4.15 The occlusal surface is partially filled as a result of compression forces vectoring the cement upward against the taper of the abutment

Abutment Modifications and Cement Flow: Occlusal Venting Effect and the Internal Vented Abutment

One concept recently developed is leaving the screw access chamber open without sealing it off. This provides a reservoir for excess cement to be retained within the crown abutment system, rather than having excess cement be extruded out of the crown margin. This is beneficial from several aspects:

1. Less cement extrusion may reduce the potential for cement induced peri-implant disease.
2. Clean-up of a reduced amount of cement is considered easier and faster.
3. There is the ability to improve retentive capabilities, as the surface area of the cement contact area with the abutment is increased.

Using the abutment screw chamber as a reservoir has been studied and proven to reduce the amount of cement extruded out of the crown abutment margin, as well as change the retention capabilities of the cement used. One other feature that has also been looked into is modifying the abutment by placing vent holes internally. The internal vent abutment (IVA) (Fig. 4.17) has two holes, 180° apart, approximately 3 mm below the occlusal surface. It has the added advantage of changing the way cement flows to enhance the amount of cement kept within the abutment compared to keeping the chamber open (Figs. 4.18 and 4.19a, b). With such modifications as the IVA, cement flow can be modified simply, which can also increase the retentive capabilities of a given cement and reduce residual cement extrusion when compared to closing off the abutment (CA) or leaving it open (OA) (Fig. 4.20).

When considering the IVA, the vent holes should only be placed in materials that are not

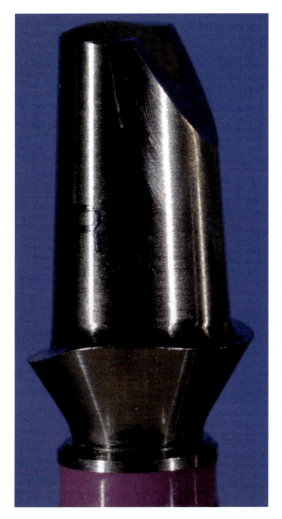

Fig. 4.16 Example of abutment that has closed off abutment screw access holes, as advocated by US dental schools

weakened by the inclusions and, therefore, are not recommended for zirconia or ceramic abutment materials. The number and sites of the vents required is currently being evaluated; presently it is considered two vents, 180° apart, with one at the mesial aspect of the implant, one at the distal, and 3 mm from the occlusal surface are adequate. Further study may be required to optimize their position. The screwhead should always be protected by a spacer to prevent cement getting into the screwdriver engagement site. Currently, the recommended material is polytetrafluoroethylene (PTFE) tape. The material can be sterilized and is easy to manipulate,

radiopaque, and less associated with malodor when retrieved.

When the Internal Vent Hole Abutment Is Not Applicable

The concept of using a modified abutment that directs cement flow internally and within the screw access channel is appealing. Not only does this help reduce the amount of cement extruded, it can also alter the retention of the crown. However, placing holes within the walls may weaken some materials, for example, ceramic abutments, zirconia abutments, or thin-metal-walled abutments. An alternative method for directing the cement within the screw access channel is by the addition of an abutment insert. The idea was derived by evaluating how fluids (in this case air is considered a fluid) can be directed by a conical device, such as a nose cone on an aircraft propeller (Fig. 4.21).

The initial stage of evaluating use of an implant abutment was done with the same form of abutments used in the internal vented cone experiment. A conical insert was fabricated from auto-curing acrylic that inserted directly into the screwhead (Fig. 4.22a–c).

Studies by the authors comparing the abutment insert indicated that the cement could be directed internally and the effects on retention where significantly different compared to closing off the abutment and leaving it open without an insert (Fig. 4.23a, b).

By evaluating and comparing the retention values of restoration using different abutment modifications, open, closed, internal vent abutment, and internal cone, a comparison graph was produced (Fig. 4.24). Once analyzed, it was noted that there was no significant difference between the internal vented abutment and the abutment insert; both were superior compared with leaving the abutment open or closing off the abutment.

The results of this test indicated that the addition of the abutment insert had an effect on cement flow similar to using the subtractive technique of placing holes in the abutment walls.

A further study was then undertaken using zirconia esthetic abutments. Thirty-six

Fig. 4.17 The open screw access chamber and the internal vented abutment (IVA). Both provide a space for excess cement to flow within. The addition of the vent holes in the IVA improves both the amount of cement kept inside the system as well as the retentive tensile strength of the cemented crown

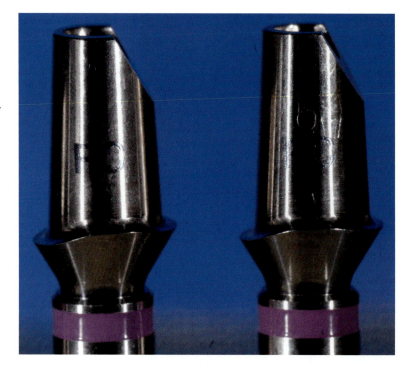

Fig. 4.18 Comparison of the amount of cement retained internally in each system. In all cases the same amount of cement was used initially

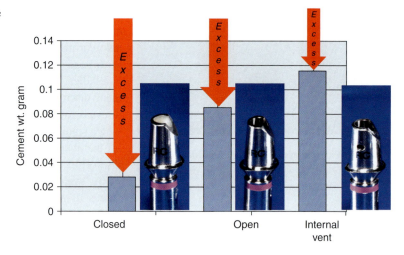

computer-aided designed and machined (CAD/CAM) anterior form zirconia abutments with conforming CAD/CAM crowns were provided by Nobel Biocare (Procera abutments). Three paired groups of 12 (one crown with one abutment) were used with the crowns cemented onto their counterpart abutment. The three groups shown in Fig. 4.25 consisted of open abutment (with a small piece of PTFE tape placed over the screwhead), a closed abutment (composite completely filling the screw channel), and an abutment insert group (an insert fabricated from a syringe tip was firmly inserted into the screwhead and projected within, but not beyond, the screw access channel).

The crowns were cemented under a load of 5 kg and maintained for 10 min until the cementing media (TempBond) had set. All crowns had

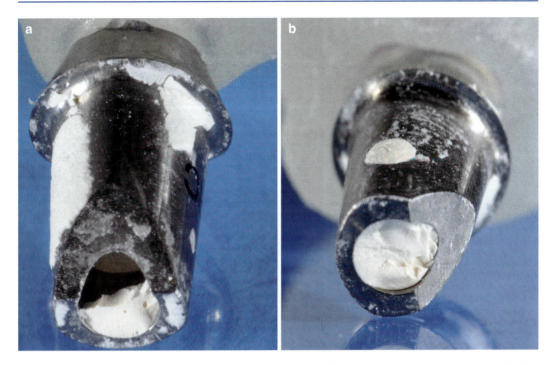

Fig. 4.19 (**a**) Cement flow was improved in the IVA compared to the (**b**) OA (open screw access) abutment, indicating more excess cement would be extruded out from the OA system

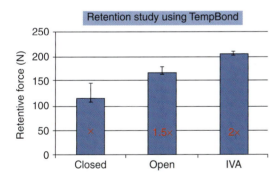

Fig. 4.20 Comparison of abutment modification and tensile retentive force to remove cemented crown. Closed was approximately half the value of the IVA

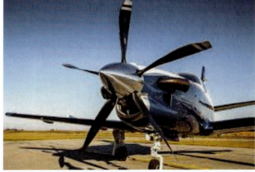

Fig. 4.21 A propeller nose cone forces air to either side and onto the blades of the prop

the same amount of cement placed within them, which represented approximately ¼ the volume of the internal of the crown (Fig. 4.26a, b).

After setting, the crown/abutment complex was cleaned of all residual excess cement from the margin, weighed, and vertical displacement height measured to ensure that the crown was fully seated. The crown and abutment were placed in 100 % humidity for 24 h, then a univer-

sal testing machine was used to apply a tensile force onto the crowns until they were displaced. The weight of the cement retained, the tensile force required to separate the crown, and the pattern of failure were all compared (Figs. 4.27a, b, 4.28a, b, and 4.29a, b).

There was no significant difference between the weight of cement retained within the open abutment or the abutment insert group, but both

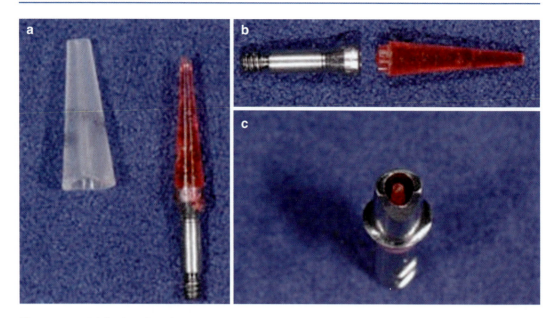

Fig. 4.22 (**a**) Fabrication of an abutment cone insert using auto-curing acrylic within a syringe tip. (**b**) The acrylic indexes the screwhead, and (**c**) when placed, it projects within the center of the screw channel

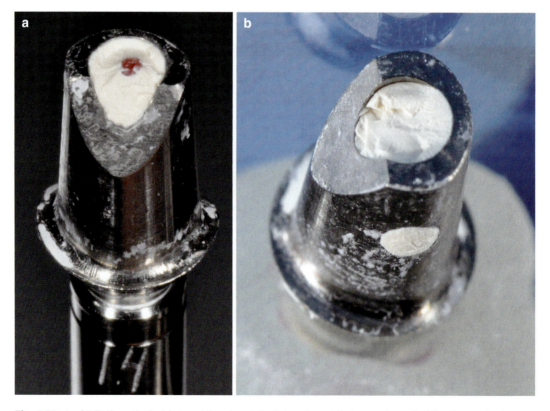

Fig. 4.23 (**a**, **b**) Both methods (abutment insert and the internal vented abutment) resulted in changes in the way cement flowed. Internalization of cement helps limit the amount extruded out of the system

Fig. 4.24 A comparison chart of the tensile forces needed to dislodge a crown related to abutment access chamber modification

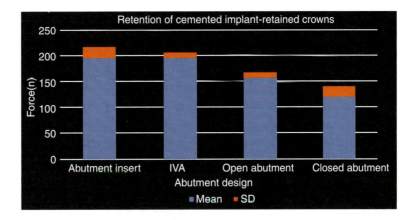

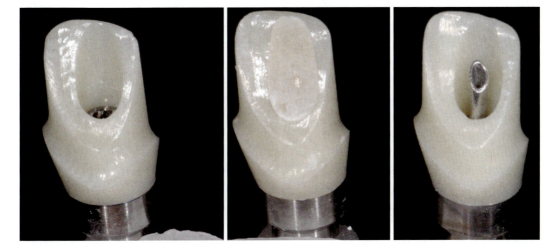

Fig. 4.25 The three groups showing modifications of the screw access channel: open, closed, and abutment insert

retained more weight than the closed group. The closed abutment failed at the lowest force (mean 108.1 N), and the pattern of cement failure was very distinctive with all the cement attached to the crown.

The results of this study concluded that cement could be directed internally and maintained within the screw channel, increasing the amount of cement within the system over closing of the screw access channel, which gave a significantly higher retention to failure value.

Clinically, where the abutment insert may be of greatest value is with short zirconia abutments with cemented crowns, such as the anterior mandibular restorations, or sites that may have greater forces placed upon them, such as maxillary canines. This

gives the clinician one more method of controlling residual excess cement, as well as a more predictable repetitive result with zirconia restorations.

Fluid Dynamics Study: Current Evaluations and Modeling of Cement Flow Within the Implant Abutment/ Crown System

Industries such as automotive, aircraft, and shipbuilding are aware of how their products behave when subjected to fluid dynamics, be it air or water. Form (shape) following function is a concept that is integral to the design of cars, airplanes, and boats. In the dental industry we commonly

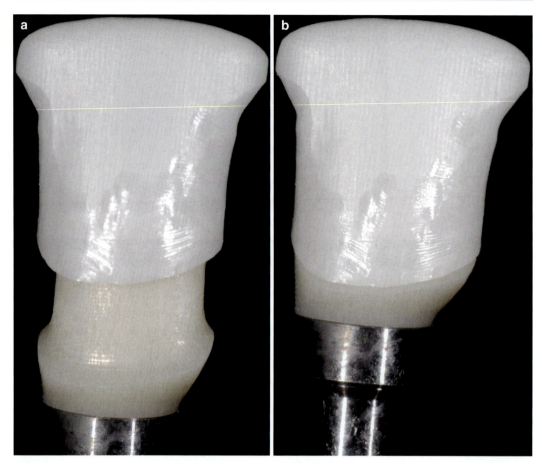

Fig. 4.26 (**a**, **b**) The CAD/CAM crowns seated onto the abutment. Note the "wings" on the crowns to allow attachment for the tensile testing device that is used to measure retention force to displacement

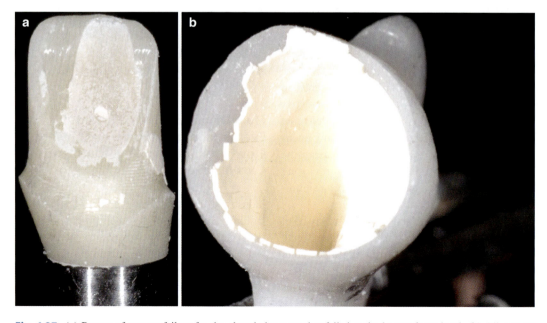

Fig. 4.27 (**a**) Pattern of cement failure for the closed abutment that failed at the lowest force level. (**b**) All cement remnants are on the crown

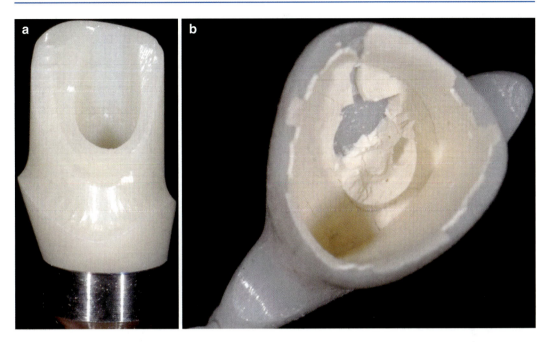

Fig. 4.28 (**a**) Cement failure with the open abutment group. Some cement is seen remaining within the abutment, which gave a slightly higher force level to failure. (**b**) An incomplete fill of the internal screw access channel of the abutment is also noted (Used with permission from Wadhwani and Chung (2014). Copyright Elsevier Inc.)

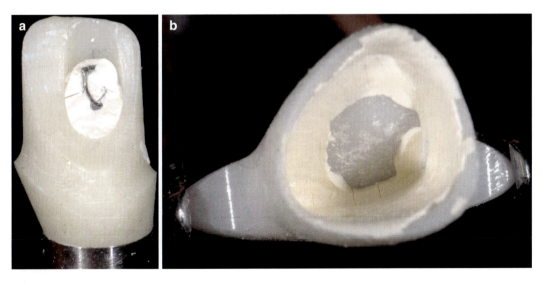

Fig. 4.29 (**a**) The abutment insert group had the highest load to failure. The cement was seen to be forced internally, and (**b**) fracture pattern showed a very different failure site compared with the other groups

use fluids, for example, when cementing implant restorations, yet we have little if any knowledge as to how these materials flow and perform as we work with them (Fig. 4.30). Form related to function is not readily considered in this fluid dynamic system, with our implant abutment shape more related to the shape we prepare teeth rather than an optimization of the cementation function.

| Group 1 | Group 2 | Group 3 |

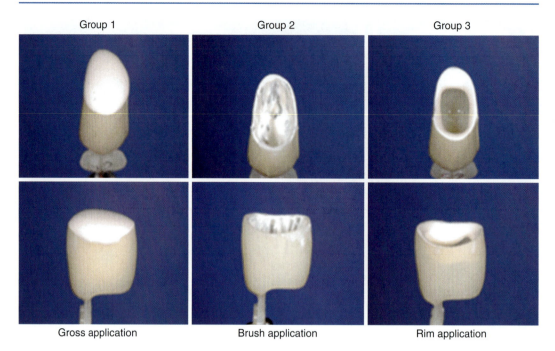

| Gross application | Brush application | Rim application |

Fig. 4.30 Clinicians do not have a good understanding of fluid dynamics, demonstrated by the amount and way they load crowns prior to cementation on implant abutments

(Used with permission from Wadhwani et al. (2012). Copyright © Quintessence Publishing Company, Inc., Chicago, IL USA)

If an understanding of how to control and optimize cement flow in the dental world were to be considered, it is likely that the form of all our cemented prosthesis would benefit. Improvements in surface contact, efficacy of the cement bond, and minimization of excess cement are to name but a few of the advantages.

We believe that the problem of peri-implant disease as it relates to cement extrusion can be addressed from a "systems control" solution. Understanding cement flow patterns, appropriate placement sites, and controlling volumes, plus changing implant designs, is key. This is only now beginning to be evaluated. This is destined to make a paradigm shift within the dental field.

Crude model systems have been used to gain an idea of cement flow, including clear plastic beakers. Implant abutments with cast crowns have also given information on how cement may work; however, using real models has restrictions. The time, number, and cost of fabricating

models for comparison to get meaningful data are immense, and controlling the variables is very complex.

Engineering simulation companies such as CD-adapco are well placed to develop methodologies for industry leaders in this field, using software solutions such as with STAR-CCM+. Computational fluid dynamic (CFD) software uses engineering simulations and provides a means of deriving data by virtual computer simulations. "Real-life" implant abutment and crown forms from scanned STL (stereo lithographic) files provide data points for the 3-D geometry. A deforming polyhedral mesh system is then developed. Relative movement simulates the crown mesh as it is placed, overlapping the mesh of the abutment, and calculations of the differences in this overlap are used (Fig. 4.31a, b). Other data input is volume to flow (VOF) which calculates how air is moved out of the system in exchange for cement at different sites. The cement is a non-Newtonian fluid so parameters from the manufacture such

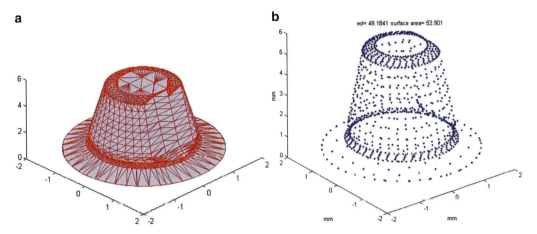

Figs. 4.31 (**a, b**) Virtual computer images produced from stereolithographic (STL) files provide the basis of this 3-D computational fluid dynamics system

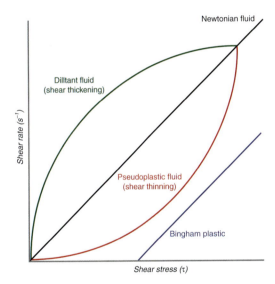

Fig. 4.32 Non-Newtonian fluid stress curves and how they relate to shear compared to Newtonian fluids. "Rheology of time independent fluids" by Chucklingcanuck—own work. Licensed under Creative Commons Attribution-Share Alike 3.0 via Wikimedia Commons—http:// commons.wikimedia.org/wiki/File:Rheology_of_time_ independent_fluids.png#mediaviewer/File:Rheology_of_ time_independent_fluids.png

as how it performs under stress and initial viscosity are used (Fig. 4.32).

With the cements used in dentistry being non-Newtonian in nature, stress has an effect on the flow of cement. For example, if you apply stress to a shear-thinning fluid by compressing

it, the fluid will flow more readily. This suggests that the force of the cement as it is squeezed increases. In cemented implant restorations, near the margins on the crown/abutment as the crown is seated, there will be a resultant increase in the rate of cement extrusion and an increase in the force of ejection. This would have an impact on adjacent soft tissues that may cause a disruption of the hemidesmosomal attachment site.

All computer simulations require validation to prove that these are real-life effects and that the variables have been adequately and correctly accounted for. This has been done with the article published in the International Journal of oral and maxillofacial Implants by Wadhwani et al. in 2011, "Effect of Implant Abutment Modification on the Extrusion of Excess Cement at the Crown-Abutment Margin for Cement-Retained Implant Restorations" (Figs. 4.33 and 4.34).

The results from the effect of abutment modification study are demonstrated in these photographs (Fig. 4.35a–c). The CFD model predicted these results, thus validating the data for this component of the analysis.

Note the prediction of the computer model and the real effect shown in this study when a vented abutment was used to modify cement flow (Fig. 4.36a, b).

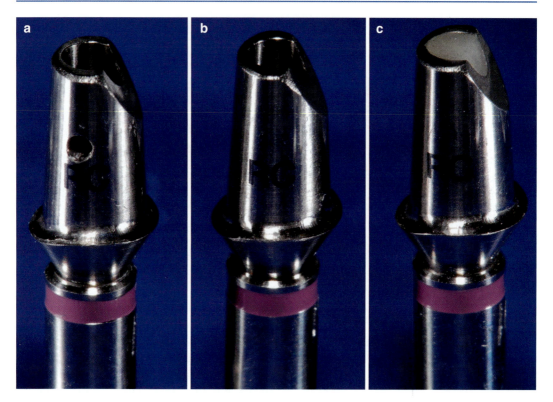

Fig. 4.33 The computer simulation were partly designed to validate the real-life study on the effects of abutment modifications. (**a**) IVA. (**b**) Open. (**c**) Closed

Simulations: Cement Application Site

Surveys of how and where dental clinicians place cement within a crown prior to seating it onto an implant abutment have indicated no standard site exists. Some place cement near to the occlusal surface, others at or near the margin of the crown.

Figure 4.37a–c can be used to show the amount (volume fraction) of cement as well as give an indication of the force of extrusion of cement when reduced to a cross section, below, which is represented by turbulence of the cement. Figure 4.38a–e shows cross-sectional frames which evaluate how the differences may affect seating and cement extrusion. Figure 4.39 represents the color gradient, and Fig. 4.40 shows a close-up of the crown margin area.

The data in the simulations does not include the soft tissues, which would tend to resist this flow if

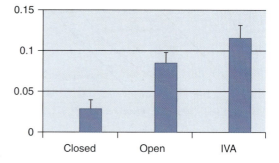

Fig. 4.34 Graph indicating that more cement is held within the system when the internal venting abutment (IVA) is used (Used with permission from Wadhwani et al. (2012). Copyright © Quintessence Publishing Company, Inc., Chicago, IL USA)

the margin lies beneath the cement lute line. It is likely that the soft tissue would result in a further increase in cement pressure at this site compared to unimpeded extrusion where no tissue exists.

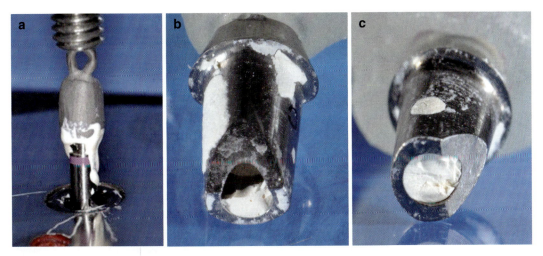

Fig. 4.35 (a–c) In vitro study evaluated the amount of cement used and flow in these abutments

Figure 4.41a–e shows cement placed in the occlusal half of the crown. As the crown is seated, a larger column of cement exists in the occlusal space compared with cement placed near the margin. The resultant flow differs with how air exchange will occur as well as the force of extrusion, which is seen much earlier, even before the crown fully seats. The final seat (Fig. 4.42) shows an incomplete margin seal and also a greater extrusion site.

The speed at which the crown is seated also affects cement flow and extrusion patterns. Figures 4.43a–c and 4.44b, c show how the speed of seating a crown affects cement flow. These images indicate that the crown should not be seated too rapidly if a seal is to be maintained and that less turbulence (mixing of cement and airflow) occurs at moderate to slow speed.

Abutment Modifications

Abutment modification simulations leaving the abutment open and abutment venting have also been evaluated, as shown in Figs. 4.45 and 4.46a, b. Areas of interest are the ability to fill the internal screw access chamber and the effect at the margin of the crown with cement extrusion. Again, with the non-Newtonian properties of cement extrusion forces when the occlusal half is loaded in preference to the apical half results in more cement force (seen by turbulence) at the margin (Fig. 4.47a, b).

The effect of overloading or underloading the crown has also been evaluated, with too much cement causing an increase force at the cement margin, yet resulting in an incomplete fill of a screw access hole when internal venting is used. Figure 4.48 shows the difference in flow patterns related to cement volume.

Conclusion

The future of implant abutment design will be predicated by the way abutments function. Restorations, abutments, and cement flow will be considered as a "system," where the whole is greater than the sum of the individual parts. With the cemented abutment, the shape, cement finish line, lute space, and all other dimensions will be subject to computational testing and design, the foremost of which will be fluid dynamics and how cement flows. The future of dental implant design will no longer be predicated on tooth shape; with form following function, it is likely the abutments of the future will look very different from what we see today.

Fig. 4.36 (**a**) Abutment modification start of simulation. (**b**) Completion of seating simulation. The computer simulation closely predicted the real-life situation, though the parameters for the real study were not controlled for speed of crown seating

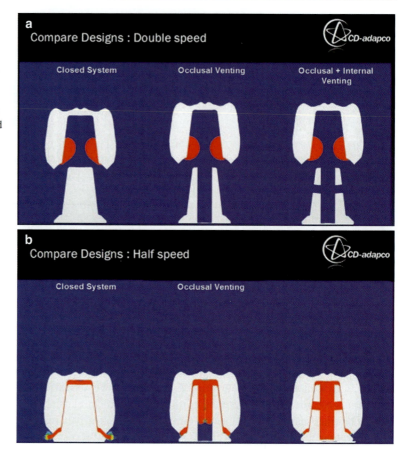

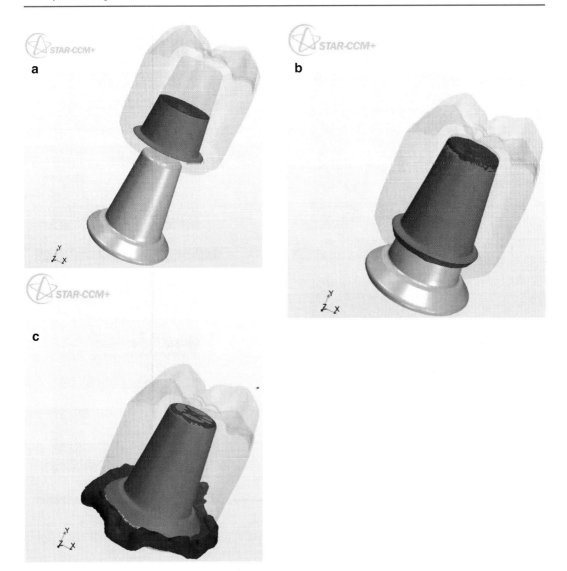

Fig. 4.37 (**a–c**) Clip images from 3-D animation of the crown seating on the abutment and resultant cement flow: (**a**) start; (**b**) 3/4 seat; (**c**) full seat with cement extrusion

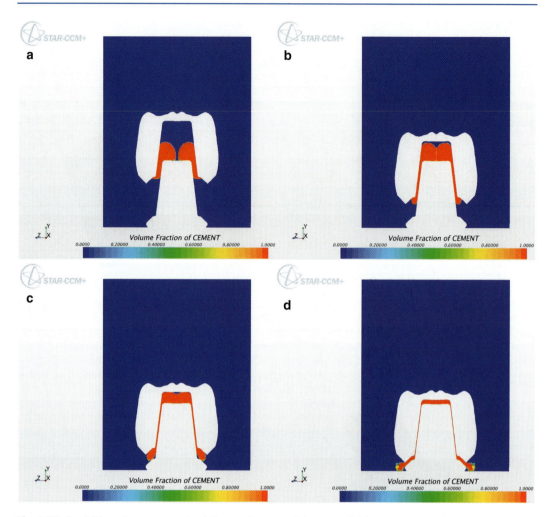

Fig. 4.38 (**a–e**) These five cross-sectional frames show how cement flows when a 1/2 toroid (a circumferential bead) of cement is placed near the margin of the crown and then seated. Blue color represents 100 % air; the red is 100 % cement. Color gradient beneath images (**b-e**) indicate mixed proportions of air/cement

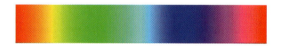

Fig. 4.39 Color gradient. Cement: air proportion exchange

Fig. 4.40 Enlargement of the crown margin area. Note the difference in coloration with the fluid fraction changes

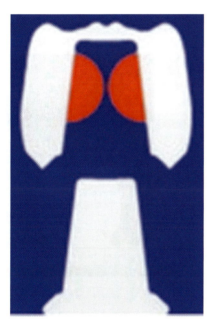

Fig. 4.41 (**a–e**) Cross-sectional frames for cement placed in the occlusal half of the crown

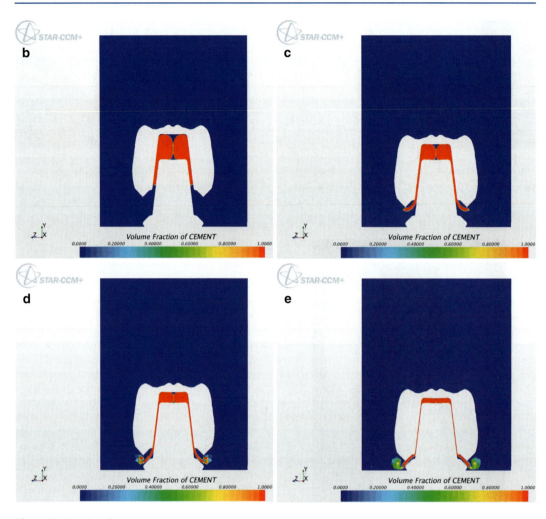

Fig. 4.41 (continued)

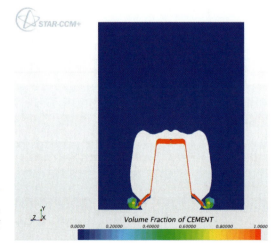

Fig. 4.42 Compared with cement placed at the crown margin, cement seal is incomplete and more turbulence of cement is noted

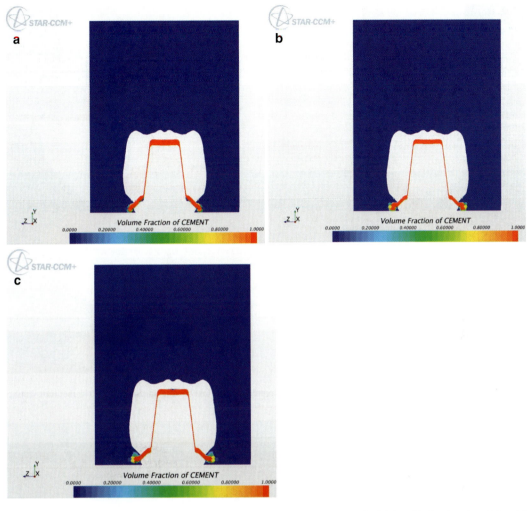

Figs. 4.43 How speed of seating affects flow. (**a**) Crown seated on abutment in 0.25 s. (**b**) Seating time 0.5 s. (**c**) Seating accomplished in 1 s. (Note the difference in cement fill at margin and occlusal sites)

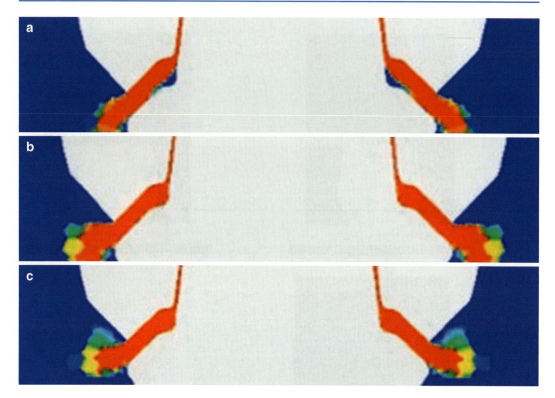

Figs. 4.44 Enlargement of the margin site and extrusion patterns at (**a**) fast seating speed (0.25 s), (**b**) medium seating speed (0.5 s), and (**c**) slow seating speed (1 s)

Fig. 4.45 All designs fill up internal space with cement before cement is extruded. Occlusal venting and internal venting greatly reduce the amount of excess cement that is extruded in the surrounding gum. Venting changes the flow of cement and may be beneficial to control the flow of cement under certain conditions, such as when air bubbles get trapped

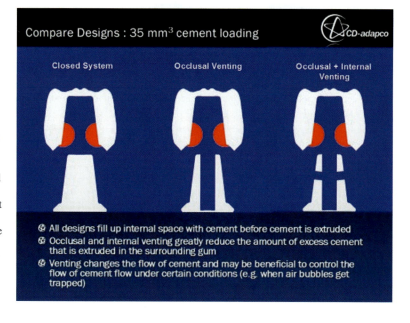

Figs. 4.46 (**a, b**) Evaluating
how cement flows with an
internal vented abutment
when the cement is applied at
different sites

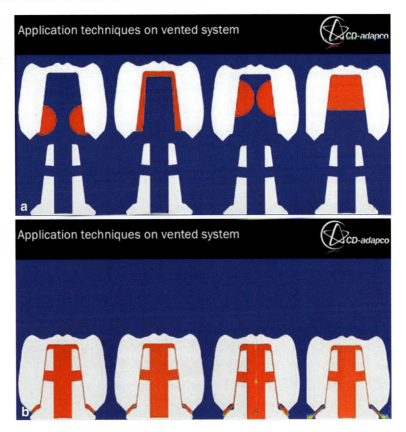

Figs. 4.46 (**a, b**) Evaluating how cement flows with an internal vented abutment when the cement is applied at different sites

Fig. 4.47 How the site of loading affects the Internal abutment insert (cone). (**a**) Cement placed as 1/2 toroid at the margin site of the crown. (**b**) Cement placed as 1/2 toroid same volume as (**a**) but higher (more occlusal) within the crown. Note how the cement has more completely filled cone insert model when cement is loaded at the margin site (**c**). Incomplete infill occurs when cement is more occlusally placed (**d**)

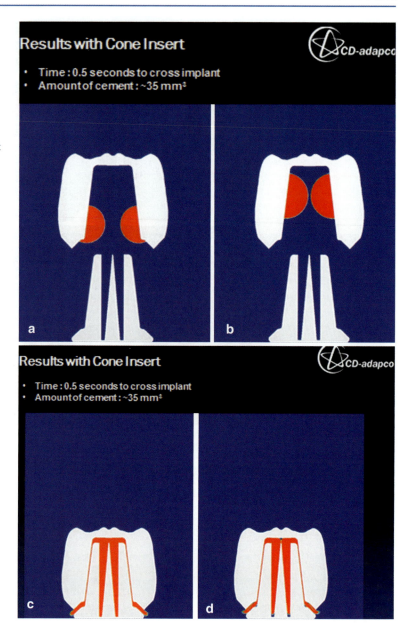

Fig. 4.48 Differences in flow pattern related to the volume of cement used in an internal vented abutment. From left to right: too little; ideal; too much

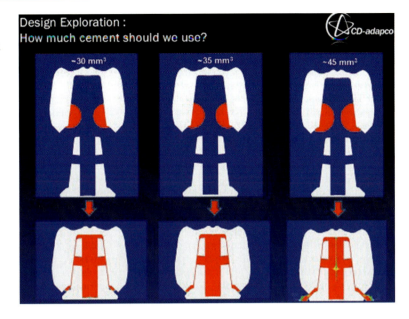

Bibliography

Arvand A, Hormes M, Reul H. A validated computational fluid dynamics model to estimate hemolysis in a rotary blood pump. Artif Organs. 2005;29:531–40.

Assif D, Rimer Y, Aviv I. The flow of zinc phosphate cement under a full-coverage restoration and its effect on marginal adaptation according to the location of cement application. Quintessence Int. 1987;18:765–74.

Beun S, Bailly C, Devaux J, Leloup G. Rheological properties of flowable resin composites and pit and fissure sealants. Dent Mater. 2008;24:548–55.

Beun S, Bailly C, Dabin A, Vreven J, Devaux J, Leloup G. Rheological properties of experimental Bis-GMA/TEGDMA flowable resin composites with various macrofiller/microfiller ratio. Dent Mater. 2009;25:198–205.

Boutsioukis C, Lambrianidis T, Kastrinakis E. Irrigant flow within a prepared root canal using various flow rates: a computational fluid dynamics study. Int Endod J. 2009;42:144–55.

Brezzi F, Lipnikov K, Simoncini V. A family of mimetic finite difference methods on polygonal and polyhedral meshes. Math Models Methods Appl Sci. 2005;15:1533–53.

Cardoso M, Torres MF, Rego MR, Santiago LC. Influence of application site of provisional cement on the marginal adaptation of provisional crowns. J Appl Oral Sci. 2008;16:214–8.

Gao Y, Haapasalo M, Shen Y, Wu H, Li B, Ruse ND, Zhou X. Development and validation of a three-dimensional computational fluid dynamics model of root canal irrigation. J Endod. 2009;35:1282–7.

Hebel KS, Gajjar R. Cement-retained versus screw-retained implant restorations: achieving optimal occlusion and esthetics in implant dentistry. J Prosthet Dent. 1997;77:28–35.

Hirt CW, Nichols BD. Volume of fluid (VOF) method for the dynamics of free boundaries. J Comput Phys. 1981;39:201–25.

Lee JH, Ulm CM, Lee IB. Rheological properties of resin composites according to variations in monomer and filler composition. Dent Mater. 2006;22:515–26.

Moráguez OD, Belser UC. The use of polytetrafluoroethylene tape for the management of screw access channels in implant-supported prostheses. J Prosthet Dent. 2010;103:189–91.

Oliva RA, Lowe JA, Ozaki MM. Film thickness measurements of a paint-on die spacer. J Prosthet Dent. 1988;60:180–4.

Patel D, Invest JCF, Tredwin CJ, Setchell DJ, Moles DR. An analysis of the effect of a vent hole on excess cement expressed at the crown-abutment margin for cement-retained implant crowns. J Prosthodont. 2009;18:54–9.

Rosenstiel SF, Land MF, Crispin BJ. Dental luting agents: a review of the current literature. J Prosthet Dent. 1998;80:280–301.

Schwedhelm ER, Lepe X, Aw TC. A crown venting technique for the cementation of implant-supported crowns. J Prosthet Dent. 2003;89:89–90.

Snjaric D, Carija Z, Braut A, Halaji A, Kovacevic M, Kuis D. Irrigation of human prepared root canal–ex vivo based computational fluid dynamics analysis. Croat Med J. 2012;53:470–9.

Tang HS, Kalyon DM. Estimation of the parameters of Herschel–Bulkley fluid under wall slip using a combination of capillary and squeeze flow viscometers. Rheologica Acta. 2004;43:80–8.

Tarica DY, Alvarado VM, Truong ST. Survey of United States dental schools on cementation protocols for implant crown restorations. J Prosthet Dent. 2010;103(2):68–79.

Taylor TD, Agar JR. Twenty years of progress in implant prosthodontics. J Prosthet Dent. 2002;88:89–95.

Tokuda Y, Song MH, Ueda Y, Usui A, Akita T, Yoneyama S, Maruyama S. Three-dimensional numerical simulation of blood flow in the aortic arch during cardiopulmonary bypass. Eur J Cardiothorac Surg. 2008;33:164–7.

Wadhwani CP, Chung K-H. The role of cements in dental implant success, part 2. Dent Today. 2013;32:46–51.

Wadhwani C, Chung K-H. Effect of modifying the screw access channels of zirconia implant abutment on the cement flow pattern and retention of zirconia restorations. J Prosthet Dent. 2014;112:45–50.

Wadhwani C, Schwedhelm R. The role of cements in dental implant success, part 1. Dent Today. 2013;32:74–9.

Wadhwani C, Hess T, Faber T, Piñeyro A, Chen CS. A descriptive study of the radiographic density of implant restorative cements. J Prosthet Dent. 2010;103:295–302.

Wadhwani C, Pineyro A, Hess T, Zhang H, Chung K-H. Effect of implant abutment modification on the extrusion of excess cement at the crown-abutment margin for cement-retained implant restorations. Int J Oral Maxillofac Implants. 2011;26:11241–6.

Wadhwani C, Hess T, Pineyro A, Opler R, Chung K-H. Cement application techniques in luting implant-supported crowns: a quantitative and qualitative survey. Int J Oral Maxillofac Implants. 2012;27:859–64.

Wadhwani C, Hess T, Pineyro A, Chung K-H. Effects of abutment and screw access channel modification on dislodgement of cement-retained implant-supported restorations. Int J Prosthodont. 2013;26:54–6.

Wadhwani C, Goodwin S, Chung K-H. Cementing an implant crown: a novel measurement system using computational fluid dynamics approach. Clin Impl Dent Relat Res. 2014; (EPub ahead of print).

Wiskott HWA, Belser UC, Scherrer SS. The effect of film thickness and surface texture on the resistance of cemented extracoronal restorations to lateral fatigue loading. Int J Prosthodont. 1999;12:255–62.

Residual Excess Cement Detection

5

Chandur P.K. Wadhwani and Thomas D. Faber

Abstract

Residual excess cement detection is mandatory if the material is to be entirely removed. Luting cement formulations do not always account for this need, with some cements colored pink so camouflaging in with the soft tissue surroundings. Detection of excess cement with radiography is also limited with many of the cements currently available. The peripheral eggshell effect is a characteristic frequently encountered when the cement is visible on a radiograph. How patterns develop and how they relate on a radiograph to the radiodensity of the cement used will assist the clinician in cement selection as well as detection. The lack of ability to find excess cement is not limited to dentistry; orthopedic medicine has also failed to understand cement flow and detection that has also resulted in failures.

Introduction

Survey data from clinicians has indicated that most dentists apply far in excess of the amount of cement required. When the restoration is fully seated, this excess must be extruded out of the abutment/crown system. Where this occurs at subgingival sites, it must be detected and adequately removed so as not to cause issues.

C.P.K. Wadhwani, BDS, MSD (✉)
Department of Restorative Dentistry, University of Washington School of Dentistry, Seattle, WA, USA

Private Practice Limited to Prosthodontics, 1200, 116th Ave NE #A, Bellevue, WA 98004, USA
e-mail: cpkw@uw.edu

T.D. Faber, DDS, MSD
Department of Periodontics, University of Washington School of Dentistry, Seattle, WA, USA

The cement type plays a vital role in the ability to allow for both detection and removal. This is not as straightforward as it appears. Some cements have been manufactured to represent gingival shading for natural esthetics—in essence they are made "pink." This increases the likelihood that they will NOT be detected visually and has presented some great issues with peri-implant disease (Figs. 5.1 and 5.2a, b).

Cement removal may also be compounded by some cement formulations being adhesive to titanium. In 1997, Agar reported on the inability to completely remove some resin cements from implant surfaces that were machined smooth. The newer resin-based cements produced today that are intended for universal use are extremely adhesive, making removal even more problematic. Coupled with the new implant surfaces that are predominantly rough, a greater tendency will exist for cement to remain (Fig. 5.3).

Radio-Opacity of Cements

As previously mentioned, residual excess cement can be the initiating factor for peri-implant disease. Being able to detect it and remove it are imperative for tissue health surrounding the implant. Techniques have been described for locating the excess cement around implant restorations with the use of a dental endoscope or, more invasively, with open flap debridement, which allows direct observation. Radiographic examination is less invasive and has been shown to be useful in the identification of cement overhangs associated with tooth-supported restora-

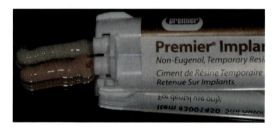

Fig. 5.1 This cement manufacturer boasts "..tasteless, odorless cement that also provides esthetic gingival shading for natural esthetics." In essence, this cement camouflages beneath the tissues and would be difficult to visually detect

tions. Recommendations have been made with respect to radiodensity levels of dental materials used to restore or cement restorations on teeth.

Comparing Implant-Specific Cements

A variety of cements are currently available for restorative procedures. Most are primarily designed for use with teeth and may be classified according to physical properties, material content, and the purpose for which they were designed, for example, interim, provisional, or definitive. Some cements have unique properties such as adhesion to tooth tissue, anticaries activity, and ion exchange. Implant-specific cements have also been formulated with useful properties relevant to implants, such as adherence to metal abutments, ease of removal of excess cement, and retrievability. Either implant-specific cements or traditional restoration cements may be used for cementing implant restorations. These cements have been extensively assessed in terms of mechanical properties, including retention capabilities, when used for implant procedures. Cement has also been shown to extrude at the implant abutment interface when subgingival margins are present. One study reported on the ease of excess cement removal as well as the damage caused to the titanium abutments by various instruments used in the process.

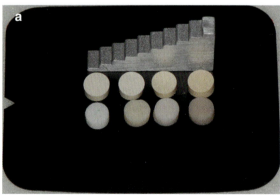
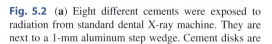
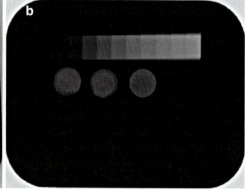

Fig. 5.2 (**a**) Eight different cements were exposed to radiation from standard dental X-ray machine. They are next to a 1-mm aluminum step wedge. Cement disks are 1 mm thick. (**b**) Only three cements are clearly visible (Reprinted from Wadhwani et al. (2010). Copyright © 2010, with permission from Elsevier)

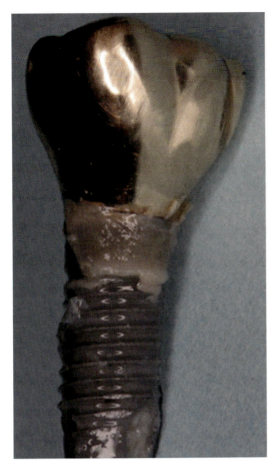

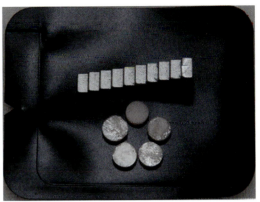

Fig. 5.4 Specimen disks with modified step wedge

Fig. 5.3 This crown was cemented with a resin-modified glass ionomer cement. It is hard and adhesive. The surface of the implant is roughened. Removal of the cement even when detected presents issues

Previous to our report, there had been no reports specific to the radiographic characteristics of cements used for implant restorations. Selection of cements should involve knowledge of the ability to detect excess cement; it is also important that a clinician be able to confirm that the cemented units are correctly positioned. Both the presence of excess cement and correct positioning could potentially be determined by non-invasive radiographic examination, provided materials in question show the appropriate radiographic density (radiodensity). Several factors may affect the radiodensity of cements; composition is probably the most significant. In addition, the material thickness, exposure settings, angulation of the X-ray beam, and the methodology used for evaluation have all been documented as factors. Radiographic images made from X-ray exposure of a digital receptor produce a spatial distribution of picture elements or pixels. Each pixel has an associated pixel value or number that ranges from 0 to 255 for an 8-bit image. The pixel value may be translated into brightness or gray level, which can be recorded and measured and is representative of radiographic density.

Our study evaluated and compared, using gray level values, the radiodensity of eight cements commonly used for implant cementation procedures. Two thicknesses of cement were compared for threshold gray levels. Disks 5 mm in diameter and 1 and 2 mm in thickness were made and radiographic images taken. Their gray levels were compared to that of a reference aluminum step wedge to determine an equivalent thickness of aluminum for the cement sample (Figs. 5.4 and 5.5). The cements that were compared are shown below in Table 5.1.

Results

Images of two cement samples are shown in Fig. 5.6a, b. Each image contains five disks of a specific cement and an aluminum step wedge as a reference, but the images in Fig. 5.6b are not visible due to the cement being poorly radio-opaque.

The specimens were ordered based on radiodensity, from highest to lowest gray level values distinguishable from the background. A comparison to the aluminum step wedge standard was recorded. The effect of changing exposure settings from 70 to 60 kVp with preset times to evaluate contrast changes was also recorded. Table 5.2 compares the aluminum equivalent thickness as found for 2-mm-thick and 1-mm-thick specimens at different exposure settings (2 mm at 70 kVp for 0.32 s, 1 mm at 70 kVp for 0.32 s, and 1 mm at 60 kVp for 0.63 s).

Of the eight cements evaluated, the highest gray level values were recorded for the zinc-containing materials (TBO, TBN, FL), which was expected due to zinc's high atomic number and electron density. In contrast, DY, which is composed of calcium hydroxide, had a lower gray level value. The zinc-containing cements

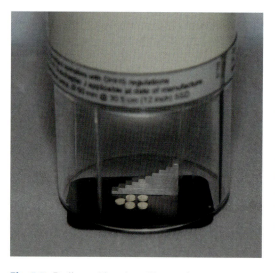

Fig. 5.5 Radiographic unit and image plate

may also offer other advantages. They may be either interim, such as the TBO and TBN varieties tested, or definitive, as is FL, allowing a choice of cement retention capabilities. The glass ionomers and resin cements are expected to have poor radiodensity properties unless specific radiopacifiers are added during formulation. This was reflected in the specimens, with RXL and RXU demonstrating less radiodensity than DY, with a lower gray level value. IM could only be detected in the 2-mm-thick specimens, indicating a lower radiodensity than either RXL or RXU. PIC was indistinguishable from the background with the imaging system used. The use of the resins and glass ionomer specimens selected can be considered problematic, as some excess material may occasionally be left in the implant soft tissue sulcus. If the tangential thickness (Fig. 5.4) is less than 1 mm, then cements RXL, RXU, or IM would be difficult, if not impossible, to detect by radiographic means.

In late 2011, Premier was reformulated to be more radio-opaque. We retested it along with other implant-specific cements. The Premier Implant Cement was the only cement in common with the previous test. Testing was done similarly to above, with cement disks being made that were again 2 mm thick and 5 mm in diameter.

Eight implant-specific cements evaluated were Premier Implant Cement (PIC), Premier Implant Cement modified with radiopacifiers (PICM), Multilink Implant shade MO0 (MI0), Multilink Implant shade MO1 (MI1), Multilink Implant shade Transparent (MIT), Implantlink Semi (ILS), Retrieve (R), and Improv (IM) (see Table 5.3). Specimen disks, 2 and 1 mm in thickness, were radiographed. Images were made

Table 5.1 Cements evaluated

Commercial name	Manufacturer	Type
Dycal (DY)	Dentsply Intl., York, PA	Calcium hydroxide
Fleck's (FL)	Mizzy Inc., Cherry Hill, NJ	Zinc phosphate
Improv (IM)	Alvelogro, Snoqualmie, WA	Resin
Premier Implant Cement (PIC)	Premier Products Co., Plymouth Meeting, PA	Resin
RelyX Luting (RXL)	3 M ESPE, St. Paul, MN	Glass ionomer
RelyX Unicem (RXU)	3 M ESPE, St. Paul, MN	Universal resin
TempBond Original (TBO)	Kerr Corp., Orange, CA	Zinc oxide/eugenol
TempBond NE (TBN)	Kerr Corp., Orange, CA	Zinc oxide/noneugenol

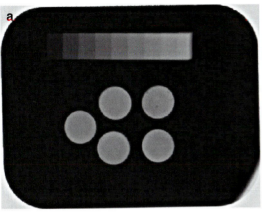

Fig. 5.6 (**a**) TempBond Original, 2-mm-thick specimens imaged at 70 kVp. (**b**) Premier Implant Cement, 2-mm-thick specimens imaged at 70 kVp. The cement is poorly radio-opaque, so it is not visible on the radiograph (Reprinted from Wadhwani et al. (2010). Copyright © 2010, with permission from Elsevier)

Table 5.2 Results: radiographic aluminum (mm) equivalence values for cements

Material	2-mm specimen, 70 kVp	1-mm specimen, 70 kVp	1-mm specimen, 60 kVp
TBO	8.11	4.52	4.53
TBN	7.13	3.65	3.64
FL	6.58	3.53	3.54
DY	3.78	1.39	ND
RXU	2.88	ND	ND
RXL	2.58	ND	ND
IM	2.29	ND	ND
PIC	ND	ND	ND

TBO TempBond Original, *TBN* TempBond NE, *FL* Fleck's, *DY* Dycal, *RXU* RelyX Unicem, *RXL* RelyX Luting, *IM* Improv, *PIC* Premier Implant Cement, *ND* Not detected

Table 5.3 Implant-specific cements compared, including the reformulated Premier Implant Cement

Commercial name	Manufacturer	Type
Premier Implant Cement (PIC)	Premier Products Co. Plymouth Meeting, Pa	Resin cement
Premier Implant Cement with Modifier (PICM)	Premier Products Co. Plymouth Meeting, Pa	Resin cement
Multilink Implant "Zero" "Third Cement" (MI0)	Ivoclar Vivadent Inc. Amherst, NY	Resin cement
Multilink Implant (MI1)	Ivoclar Vivadent Inc. Amherst, NY	Resin cement
Multilink Implant Transparent (MIT)	Ivoclar Vivadent Inc. Amherst, NY	Resin cement
Implantlink Semi (ILS)	DETAX GmbH & Co. KG Ettlingen, Germany	Resin cement
Retrieve (R)	Parkell Inc. Edgewood, NY	Resin cement
Improv (IM)	Alvelogro, Snoqualmie, WA	Resin

using photostimulable phosphor (PSP) plates with standardized exposure values. Again average gray level value representative of radiodensity for each of the seven cements were compared and referenced to a standard aluminum step wedge. An equivalent thickness of aluminum in millimeters was calculated using best straight line fit estimates.

Examples of the images taken are shown in Fig. 5.7a, b. Multilink Implant Cement (MI1) and the Premier Implant Cement with Modifier (PICM) are shown side by side. Note how the disks are not visible in Fig. 5.7b due to the cement's poor radio-opacity.

Table 5.4 shows the results for the 2- and 1-mm-thick disks. The gray level values obtained are represented as the equivalent thickness in aluminum for comparison. Images were taken at 70 kVp, 0.32 s, and 7 mA.

It is interesting to note that at the setting used (70 kVp, 0.32 s, and 7 mA), the modified Premier Implant Cement with Modifier was not observable. Upon changing settings to a lower kVp (60 kVp, .32 s, 7 mA), the Premier Implant Cement (PIC) and Premier Implant Cement with

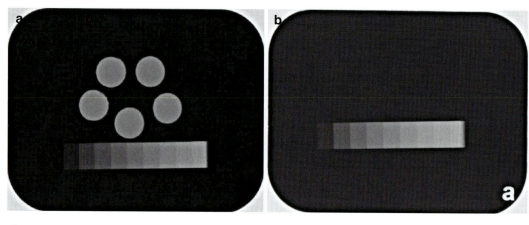

Fig. 5.7 (**a**) 2-mm-thick sample disks of Multilink Implant Cement (MI1). (**b**) Five disks made with Premier Implant Cement with Modifier (PICM) imaged at 70 kVp, 0.32 s, and 7 mA, which are not visible on the radiograph because the cement is poorly radio-opaque (Reprinted from Wadhwani et al. (2010). Copyright © 2010, with permission from Elsevier)

Table 5.4 Comparison of equivalent aluminum thicknesses for the implant-specific cements

Cement name	Equivalent aluminum thickness, mm for 2-mm-thick cement samples	Equivalent aluminum thickness, mm for 1-mm-thick cement samples
MI1	7.6	3.98
MIT	7.52	3.59
MI0	7.35	3.83
R	2.25	Not observable
IM	1.35	Not observable
ILS	Not observable	Not observable
PICM	Not observable	Not observable
PIC	Not observable	Not observable

MI1 Multilink Implant, *MIT* Multilink Implant Transparent, *MI0* Multilink Implant "Zero" "Third Cement", *R* Retrieve, *IM* Improv, *ILS*, Implantlink Semi, *PICM* Premier Implant Cement with Modifier, *PIC* Premier Implant Cement

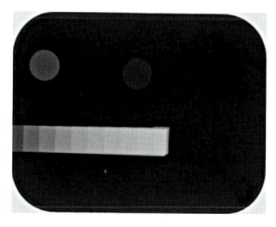

Fig. 5.8 Premier Implant Cement (PIC) above and Premier Implant Cement with Modifier (PICM) below are just observable at lower exposures settings of 60 kVp, .32 s, 7 mA

Modifier (PICM) were found to be just barely observable (Fig. 5.8).

Summary of Findings

In the above comparison of implant-specific cements, the most opaque cements were the Multilink Implant Cements MO0, MO1, and Transparent. It is worthy to note that they use fillers composed of barium glass and ytterbium trifluoride, which have higher atomic numbers of 56 and 70, respectively. These fillers compose 40 % of the cement. Much less in opaqueness is the Retrieve, which is composed of uncured acrylate and methacrylate ester monomers, benzoyl peroxide, and silane-treated glass. These resin-based cements depend on the fillers to give any radio-opaque properties.

These comparisons are done to help the restorative dentist gauge the radiographic character of the cement material used. It is desirable that the cement be as radio-opaque as possible while demonstrating other required physical properties. This should better help the dentist in choosing the appropriate cement to use. It is hoped that the manufacturers consider making cements with more radio-opaque properties.

Clinical Variations in the Ability to Detect Residual Excess Cement[1]

Residual excess cement (REC) is a common complication of cement-retained implant prostheses, which can result in a local inflammatory process, documented as a cause of peri-implant disease. The etiology is not fully understood but is believed to relate to bacterial colonization of the foreign material, which can occur several years after the restoration has been completed. If the REC is identified and removed, the majority of problems can be resolved. The prevention of cement extrusion during the restoration process beyond the restorative cement margins cannot be underestimated; however, this may be more difficult than it appears. In vitro model systems have demonstrated the difficulty in controlling and removing REC by visual and tactile means, even when supragingival crown/abutment margins have been placed. Radiographic evaluation allows for a noninvasive evaluation of the site to locate REC. Detection is influenced by factors such as the composition of the cement, the amount, and the site. Other disciplines within dentistry have required radio-opacity specifications for cements, but no mandatory minimal standard specification exists for implant cements. This clinical report highlights varying degrees of REC detection by using intraoral dental radiographs. The radiographic detection and characteristic patterns of cement flow are also described.

Clinical Reports

Patient 1, Cement Superimposition

A 48-year-old male patient in good general health presented for replacement of the maxillary right central incisor that had been extracted 6 months earlier. Initial impressions were made, followed by diagnostic waxing and the fabrication of a surgical guide. The guide was used to direct the implant placement such that the head of the implant (Standard Plus, Regular Neck, Straumann, Andover, MA) was located 3 mm below the proposed facial gingival margin. A 3-mm-high healing abutment (Straumann) was placed at the time of surgery, and an interim removable prosthesis was provided for the patient during the healing phase. Four months after the implant placement, clinical and radiographic integration was confirmed, and the patient was referred for the definitive restoration. This consisted of a metal ceramic crown, cemented with a zinc oxide and eugenol cement (TempBond, Kerr, West Collins, Orange, CA) onto a cast gold custom abutment (SynOcta gold abutment, Straumann).

Seven months after completion of the restoration, the patient presented with a draining sinus tract on the midfacial aspect of the implant site (Fig. 5.9a).

A size 20 ISO gutta percha point (Henry Schein, Melville, NY) was placed into the sinus tract (Fig. 5.9b), and a radiograph was made. The gutta percha point terminated at the abutment/ crown interface (Fig. 5.9c). Initial nonsurgical attempts to debride the site under local anesthesia were unsuccessful, and it was decided to treat the area surgically. Full-thickness facial and lingual flaps were elevated to reveal residual subgingival REC deposits at the crown/abutment interface (Fig. 5.9d). The REC was located predominantly on the facial aspect, such that the superimposition of the cement on the metal implant components rendered the cement almost impossible to detect radiographically.

The residual cement was removed with hand scalers (Implantcare tip currettes: Columbia 4r/4 l, 204 s, h6/h7, Hu-Friedy, Rockwell, IL

[1] Reproduced with kind permission from the *Journal of Prosthetic Dentistry*—Author Wadhwani CPK, 2010

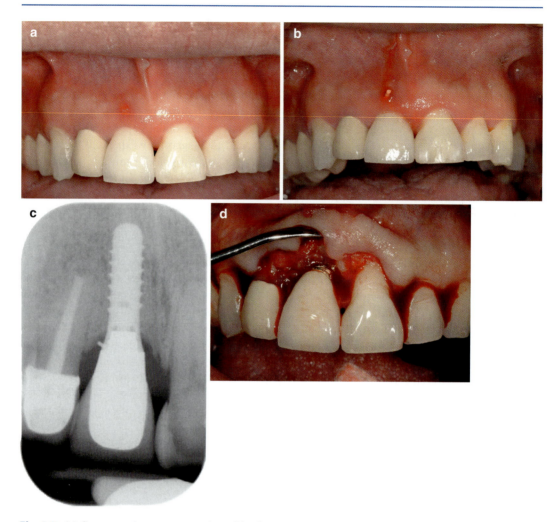

Fig. 5.9 (**a**) Seven months post-cementation of implant crown. (**b**) Gutta percha point placed into sinus tract. (**c**) Radiograph, gutta percha point visible. (**d**) Full-thickness flap raised, exposing cement residue

USA), taking care to avoid damaging the implant surface. An autogenous connective tissue graft was harvested from the right palatal vault area and secured over the facial aspect of the implant. The sinus tract resolved completely within 6 months, and the patient was placed on a 4-month interval recall program, including probing depth monitoring and annual radiographs.

Patient 2: Highly Radio-Opaque Cement

A 55-year-old woman was referred for an implant restoration to replace the maxillary left lateral incisor. The tooth had been extracted 2 years previously and replaced with a provisional removable prosthesis. The patient reported no medical problems or known allergies at the time of consultation. Clinical evaluation revealed a buccolingual concavity at the proposed implant site. Radiographically, a crestal deficiency was noted in relation to the mesial aspect of the adjacent canine. An implant (NobelSpeedy, Nobel Biocare, Yorba Linda, CA USA), shown in Fig. 5.10a, was placed together with a simultaneous addition of bone graft material—a combination of 50 % xenograft (Bio-Oss, Osteohealth, Shirley, NY USA) and 50 % allograft cortical particulate mineralized FDBA (LifeNet Health Inc. Virginia beach, VA USA) on the buccal aspect of the implant.

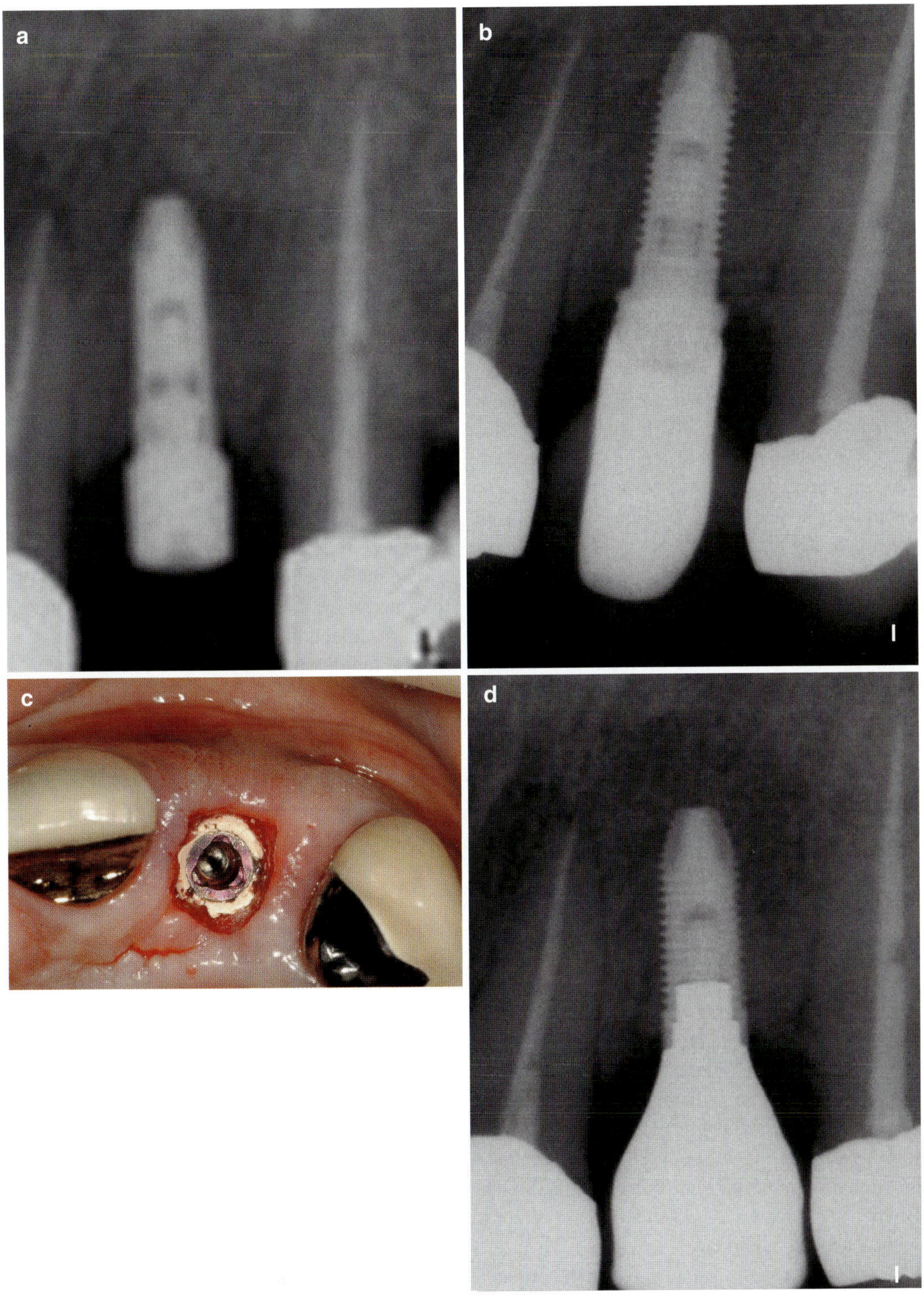

Fig. 5.10 (**a**) Pre-restoration radiograph; implant considered integrated. (**b**) Post-cementation radiograph; restoration with radio-opacity noted. (**c**) Crown and abutment removed, cement encircling abutment visible. (**d**) Post-treatment radiograph; note replacement with screw-retained restoration

The bony defect noted on the adjacent maxillary left canine was managed with the same augmentation materials. A collagen membrane (Bio-Gide, Osteohealth) and an autogenous connective tissue graft harvested from the left palate to provide additional ridge augmentation were placed over the hard tissue augmentation site. The patient continued to wear the removable provisional prosthesis for an additional month, allowing the site to heal. Once the implants had achieved clinical and radiographic osseointegration (Fig. 5.10a), the patient was referred to a restorative dentist for definitive treatment. One week after the definitive restoration was placed, the patient returned for a soft tissue and radiographic post-restoration evaluation. The soft tissue appeared pale pink with no signs of inflammation. However, a radiograph revealed the presence of REC (Fig. 5.10b). On removing the crown and the abutment, the implant platform was found to be encircled by cement (Fig. 5.10c), which was subsequently removed. A new healing abutment was placed and the restoring dentist was asked to reconsider the restorative options available. Because the implant position was favorable, the subsequent restoration was screw-retained (Fig. 5.10d), which eliminated the issues associated with cement. The patient was then provided with supportive periodontal therapy and annual implant assessment including radiographic, occlusal, and soft tissue evaluation.

Patient 3: The Circumferential Effect

A 68-year-old woman presented with a type IV fracture of the left lateral incisor. After clinical and radiographic assessment, the treatment option chosen was to extract the tooth remnant and evaluate for possible immediate implant placement. The tooth was extracted by gentle elevation, leaving an intact facial bony plate. An immediate implant (Osseotite MicroMiniplant, 3.25/3.4, Biomet 3i, Warsaw, IN USA) was placed along with a healing abutment (Fig. 5.11a). No graft material was used, as the gap between the implant and the facial bony wall was less than 2 mm. An invisible retainer (Clear Splint Biocryl 0.75 mm,

Great Lakes Orthodontics Ltd., Tonawanda, NY) containing an acrylic resin denture tooth (Trublend, Dentsply International, York, PA USA) was used for a provisional restoration. The healing was uneventful, and 10 months postoperatively, a screw-retained acrylic resin provisional crown was attached to the implant to contour the soft tissue emergence profile. It remained fixed to the implant for 6 months. The definitive restoration chosen was a metal ceramic crown, cemented onto a custom abutment (Atlantis, Astra Tech Inc., Waltham, MA USA) with resin-reinforced glass ionomer cement (Vitremer, 3 M ESPE, St. Paul, MN USA). Nine months after placement of the final restoration, the patient presented complaining of a bad taste originating at the implant area. The site was evaluated, and suppuration was expressed upon gentle finger pressure around the soft tissues adjacent to the implant. A radiograph revealed a radio-opacity immediately adjacent to the implant restoration complex with associated interproximal bone loss (Fig. 5.11b).

The radiographic appearance of the REC was indicative of a thin circumferential layer of cement, which was magnified by tangential exposure to the radiographic beam (Fig. 5.11c). The site was subsequently treated by closed debridement. The follow-up radiograph (Fig. 5.11d) and clinical examination failed to reveal residual cement, and no signs or symptoms of inflammation were detected. The patient was observed 1 month later and then at three monthly intervals for the first year. No further issues relating to the implant site were found.

Patient 4: Radiolucent Cement

A 58-year-old man with a history of colon cancer and smoking presented with failing endodontic treatment on the distal root of the mandibular left first molar. The prognosis for the tooth was hopeless and it was extracted. The extraction socket site allowed for immediate implant (Wide Neck implant, Straumann, Andover, MA USA) placement with simultaneous hard tissue allograft bone augmentation (Puros, Zimmer Dental, Carlsbad, CA USA). The platform of the implant was such

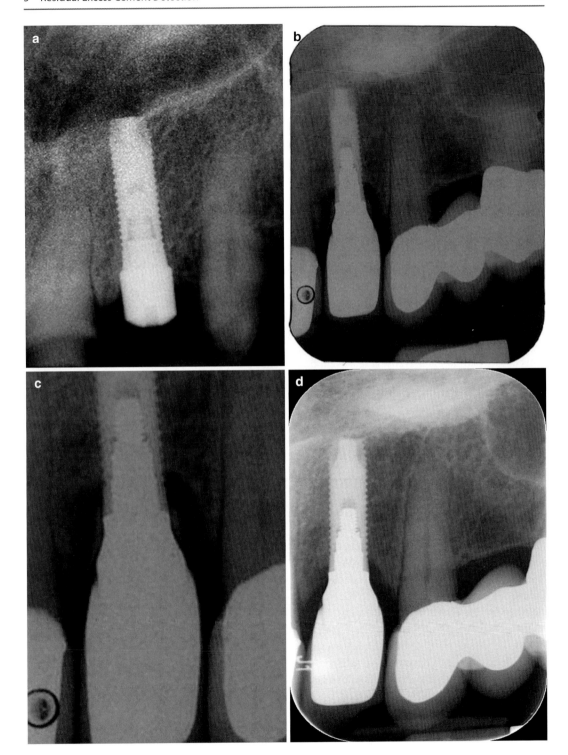

Fig. 5.11 (**a**) Pre-restoration radiograph of implant. (**b**) Radiograph indicating "peripheral eggshell" effect—layer of REC. (**c**) Magnified view of B. (**d**) Post-treatment radiograph with cement removed

that the buccal margin was placed 1 mm below the existing gingival margin. The implant site remained unrestored for 7 months with uneventful healing. Once clinical osseointegration was confirmed, a stock abutment (Wide Neck solid abutment, Straumann) was placed and a torque of 35 Ncm was applied. A closed-tray impression technique followed. A metal ceramic crown was fabricated, evaluated for fit, occlusion, and color, and then cemented with an implant-specific acrylic urethane cement (Premier Implant Cement, Premier Dental, Plymouth Meeting, PA USA). A radiograph was made after cementation to verify the complete seating of the restoration and the removal of REC. The patient was placed on a 3-month alternating hygiene schedule with the restorative dentist and periodontist. Routine peri-implant probing measurements and radiographs made 14 months after final restoration were unremarkable and had no signs or symptoms of any pathological events (Fig. 5.12a, b).

However, at 32 months after comletion of the restoration, clinical evidence of inflammation was noted: bleeding on probing, an increase in peri-implant probing depths, and a radiograph indicated bone loss associated with the implant (Fig. 5.12c). Treatment was initiated by removing the crown but leaving the stock abutment in place. The periodontist used a full-thickness flap procedure to expose the residual REC circumferentially around the implant (Fig. 5.12d). Debridement of the inflammatory tissue was performed with both hand and ultrasonic instrumentation by using a piezoelectric unit (Piezon Master 600, Electro Medical Systems, Dallas, TX USA) with a plastic-coated implant cleaning tip (PI, Piezon implant cleaning, Electro Medical Systems). The implant surface was treated with sterile saline—0.9 % sodium chloride—(Salvin Dental Specialties, Inc., Charlotte, NC USA) before grafting the residual defect with an allograft material (Puros, Zimmer, Carlsbad, CA USA). This was followed by flap closure (Fig. 5.12e).

Discussion

REC (residual excess cement) results from extrusion of cement during the restoration placement process. Factors that determine the quantity and location of the REC are beyond the scope of this report. However, they include amount of cement used, viscosity and flow properties of the cement, forces during placement, margin integrity, ability to remove unset cement, abutment material, texture, and shape.

The association of cement remnants with peri-implant diseases requires that any REC beneath the tissues around an implant be detected and removed. However, the detection and removal of REC by visual and tactile methods has been shown to be problematic even when the implant crown cement finish line height is controlled. The influence of margin location on the amount of undetected cement excess after insertion of cement-retained implant restorations was noted in a study by Linkevičius even when margins were placed 1 mm above the soft tissue level. The results of this study indicated a significant difference among each test group for all but the deepest two groups, with margin depths ranging from −3 to 1 mm above the soft tissues at 1 mm intervals. It was reported that the −2 and −3 mm level soft tissue margins showed the greatest cement excess weight of all groups. The margins of the patients reported were all 1–2 mm below their respective free gingival margins, with the exception of Patient 3, where the margin was 3 mm below.

The radiograph relating to Patient 3 also indicates the crown failed to seat completely, leaving a margin that would have allowed great excess cement to be extruded during placement. This may have occurred because of too much cement within the crown, tight proximal contact, tight fit of the crown, inadequate cement space, not following cement manufacturer recommendations regarding working and setting time, or inadequate pressure application while seating the crown. Some of these issues are seen on a pre-cementation radiograph and can be corrected before complete seating.

There are no minimum specific radiographic standards for implant cements. The radio-opacity of some commonly used cements has been documented and a large variation in radiographic detection ability has been reported. Some cements have high radiographic density, which

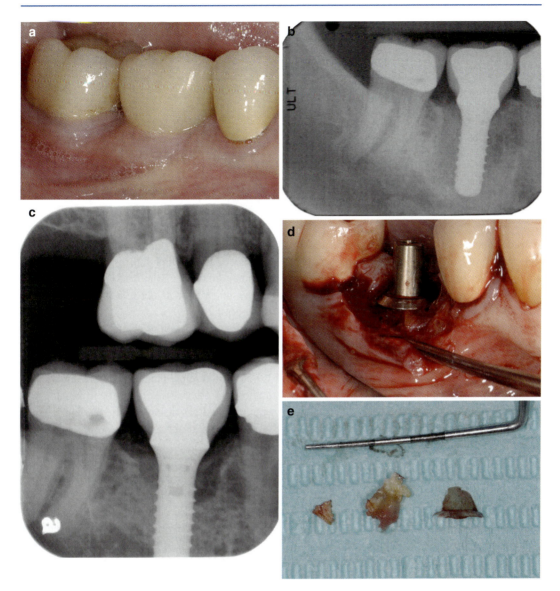

Fig. 5.12 (**a**) Post-insertion radiograph of implant placed in mandibular right first molar site. (**b**) Fourteen months post-restoration radiograph, no evidence of bone loss around implant. (**c**) Thirty-two months post-insertion radiograph, bone loss evident, no indication of residual cement. (**d**) Surgical exposure of REC. (**e**) Cement remnants removed compared to periodontal probe with 3 mm markings (Pictures Courtesy of Dr. Tim Hess)

allows for easy radiographic detection; others cannot be detected even at 2 mm thickness. The radiographic opacity of a material varies directly with the third power of the atomic number of the absorber elements. For this reason, the zinc found in zinc phosphate and zinc oxide/eugenol cements is highly detectable (Patient 2). This is in contrast to the low atomic number elements found in acrylic urethane cements that are difficult to detect radiographically (Patient 4), unless the manufacturer purposefully adds agents containing higher atomic numbers to increase the radio-opacity.

Apart from the composition of the cement, the location and pattern of cement extrusion around the restoration may alter the ability to detect the excess. Patient 1 is an example of the use of a highly radio-opaque cement (containing zinc) that

Fig. 5.13 (a) "Peripheral eggshell" effect, X-ray beam, and radiographic plate are perpendicular to cement film, exposing increased thickness of cement. *T* tangential depth, R_c radius of implant plus cement, R_i radius of Implant. (**b**) Calculation:

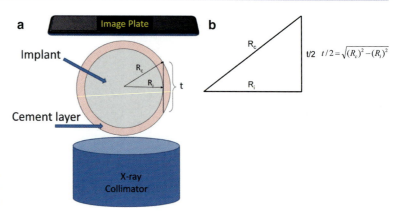

$$T = 2\sqrt{\left(R_c^2 - R_i^2\right)}$$

(Reprinted from Wadhwani et al. (2010). Copyright © 2010, with permission from Elsevier)

extruded facially to the implant surface, making detection problematic. The use of a radiographic tracer marker highlighted the origin of the tract, which, upon surgical exposure, revealed the REC.

The site of extrusion may, under the right conditions of cement flow, enhance radiographic detection. Patient 2 is an example of a cement (resin-modified glass ionomer) that is less radiopaque than a zinc cement and that was detectable even though a minimal layer was used. This is because implants are generally circular in cross section, and when the cement flow follows this shape, a circumferential layer results. Because the X-ray beam passes tangentially through the thickness of the thin cement layer (a longer path than the radial thickness of the cement), an observed attenuation results, i.e., the peripheral eggshell effect (Fig. 5.13a, b).

Differing radiographic appearances of REC extrusion into the peri-implant tissues have been demonstrated. These detection patterns are a result of the amount, site, and radiographic density of cements used.

Problems with Cement Flow and Dental Implants: Dentistry Is Not Alone

This section describes four patterns found with intraoral radiography when evaluating areas for REC. The clinical report presented demonstrates the varying degrees of radio-opacity found in cements used for implant restorations and describes the circumstances under which

the characteristic radiographic image was produced. By understanding these issues, the clinician may be able to diagnose problems earlier and better select a cement for implant restorations.

Although this text is primarily involved with the effects of residual excess cement around dental implants and their consequences, this problem is not limited to the dental field. Research by the author into other forms of medical implants that are cemented has discovered medicine may have an even larger problem.

Looking at how total hip replacements, known as total hip arthroplasty (THA), are undertaken has found some very disturbing information. A case report was published in 2009 that describes the postsurgical findings of excess cement around a replacement hip joint. The case presentation in the *Journal of Medical Case Reports 2009* (Reilingh et al. 2009) concerns a 59-year-old woman who presented with rest pain, numbness, and cramps in the operated limb after hip replacement. Cement leakage under the transverse ligament had caused occlusion of the common femoral artery, necessitating vascular reconstruction.

During surgery, it is common practice to cement both the acetabular as well as the femoral components. The acetabular component is prepared with several anchorage holes to mechanically retain the cement to the bone prior to cementation of the cup. On completion of the surgery, the limb is aligned and a radiograph is made to confirm centralization of the components (Fig. 5.14).

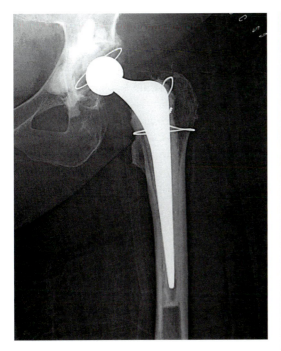

Fig. 5.14 Anteroposterior radiograph showing the cemented total hip prosthesis with no obvious common femoral artery due to cement (From Reilingh et al. (2009))

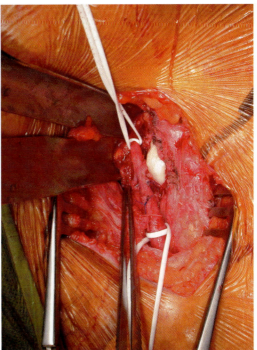

Fig. 5.15 Lesion of the posterior aspect of the cement extrusion in the pelvis or soft tissues (From Reilingh et al. (2009))

In this case, recovery was considered adequate enough to allow the patient to be discharged 10 days after surgery. Two months later, she presented in the outpatient center with excruciating rest pain, numbness, and cramps. Arterial duplex examination confirmed an occlusion of the left common femoral artery. Inguinal surgical exploration found a large mass of cement crushing the posterior aspect of the common femoral artery (Figs. 5.15, 5.16 and 5.17).

The technique of cementing implants within the femur was first popularized by Professor Sir John Charnley in 1962 and has since become one of the most common operations in the world. Most THAs are a result of arthritis causing pain to the patient. The THA involves sectioning of the femur and replacement with a tapered implant prosthesis, a "post" with a ball articulation. This seats into a "cup" placed within the acetabulum, the hip socket. The cement is introduced into the femur, using a syringe, and packed into the acetabular fossa prior to cementing the prostheses. It is clear that little control on the amount of cement used exists, again with the medical profession not

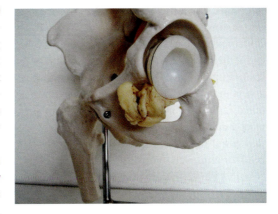

Fig. 5.16 Reconstruction of the cement leakage under the transverse ligament (From Reilingh et al. (2009))

having clear parameters for how much cement is required or how to control the flow pattern.

Studies evaluating the number of times cement was seen to extrude beyond the confines of the acetabulum have been undertaken. Using radiographic assessment, extrusion occurred in 44 % of cases. With the knowledge of the limitations of

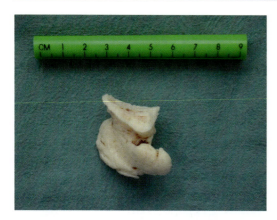

Fig. 5.17 The unique print of the cemented acetabular cup on the extracted cement mass clearly demonstrates the pathomechanism of leakage under the transverse ligament (From Reilingh et al. (2009))

radiographic assessment in a single plane, this number is likely much higher.

The major considerations for the orthopedic surgeon are viscosity of the cement, time to setting, and temperature control of the cement as it goes through an exothermic setting reaction. Another critical feature is maintaining the blood within the femur during cementation. It is understood that if insufficient pressure is exerted during seating of the femur implant, blood can contaminate the cement, causing incomplete lining of the cavity. Also, during cementation of the femur implant, an event may occur—the production of emboli. Studies have indicated with traditional seating techniques as the femur implant is placed emboli occur in 100 % of cases, which may result in death in the operating theater. The need for improved femur cementation methods is currently being investigated, but even with newer prostheses and techniques, the risk of larger emboli causing issues still occurs in 20 % of cases.

The association of bone cement and THA is known as bone cement implantation syndrome and is on the increase with more and more elderly patients requiring hip surgeries. Risk factors initially focused on the type of cement, methyl-methacrylate (a material well known to dentists!), with known issues from the monomer. This

has been shown to cause histamine release, complement activation, and endogenous cannabinoid-mediated vasodilation. Techniques in the seating of the prosthesis have also been cited as risk factors, with packing the femur with cement increasing the risk of emboli and venting the femur implant reducing the risks.

The materials used in orthopedics with THA mimic many of the limitations noted in dental implant restoration. No protocols exist. Ideal cement properties have not been elicited, so many different forms of cement with differing properties exist. Poor radiodensity, little understanding of flow properties, and little, if any, quantifying of the amount required or application technique as well as the implant design, appears rudimentary with little consideration to the cement flow.

Interestingly enough, the association of THA with dentistry is well understood by orthopedic surgeons and dentists alike, in that patients undergoing invasive forms of dental treatment including routine cleanings are given a prophylaxis antibiotic to prevent oral microbes from contaminating the artificial joint. To the authors' best knowledge, there exists no data on how well the cements used in THAs or other prosthesis behave with the microbes of the oral environment.

Conclusion

The previous chapters have described the issues related to residual excess cement and health. If the excess cement can be identified, the problem may be resolved. Characteristics of the implant shape and site, along with radiographic assessment, will improve the ability to determine where the cement may remain. The cement manufacturers must also understand the issues we as clinicians are presented with; their goal should be to assist in the identification by formulating cements that are visible, easy to find, and highly radio-opaque.

The medical world is constantly changing and trying to improve with each new challenge presented and it, too, must look into common procedures and understand how problems such as excess cement need to be addressed.

Bibliography

Abdulkarim A, Ellanti P, Motterlini N, Fahey T, O'Byrne JM. Cemented versus uncemented fixation in total hip replacement: a systematic review and meta-analysis of randomized controlled trials. Orthop Rev. 2013;5(e8):34–44.

Agar JR, Cameron SM, Hughbanks JC, Paker MH. Cement removal from restorations luted to titanium abutments with simulated subgingival margins. J Prosthet Dent. 1997;78:43–7.

Bitsch RG, Obermeyer BJ, Rieger JS, Jäger S, Schmalzried TP, Bischel OE. What is the upper limit of cement penetration for different femoral hip resurfacing components? J Arthroplasty. 2013;28:654–62.

d'Astorg H, Amzallag J, Poignard A, Roudot Thoraval F, Allain J. Periacetabular cement extrusion in the course of total hip replacement: incidence and consequences. An analysis from 269 consecutive cemented total hips. Orthop Traumatol Surg Res. 2011;97:608–14.

Donaldson AJ, Thomson HE, Harper HJ, Kenny NW. Bone cement implantation syndrome. Br J Anaesth. 2009;102:12–22.

International Organization for Standardization. ISO 4049: dentistry – polymer based restorative materials. Geneva: ISO; 2009. Available at: http://www.iso.ch/iso/en/prods-services/ISOstore/store.html.

International Organization for Standardization. ISO 6876: dental root canal sealing materials. Geneva: ISO; 2002. Available at: http://www.iso.ch/iso/en/prods-services/ISOstore/store.html.

Linkevicius T, Vindasiute E, Puisys A, Peciuliene V. The influence of margin location on the amount of undetected cement excess after delivery of cement-retained implant restorations. Clin Oral Implants Res. 2013;1:71–6.

Martin WM, Dixon JH, Sandhu H. The incidence of cement extrusion from the acetabulum in total hip arthroplasty. J Arthroplasty 2003;18(3):338–41.

Reilingh M, Hartemink KJ, Hoksbergen AW, Saouti R. Occlusion of the common femoral artery by cement after total hip arthroplasty: a case report. J Med Case Rep. 2009;3:86.

Schmidutz F, Düll T, Voges O, Grupp T, Müller T, Jansson V. Secondary cement injection technique reduces pulmonary embolism in total hip arthroplasty. Int Orthop. 2012;36:1575–81.

Wadhwani C, Hess T, Faber T, Pineyro A, Chen CSK. A descriptive study of the radiographic density of implant restorative cements. J Prosthet Dent. 2010;103(5):295–302.

Wadhwani C, Rapoport D, La Rosa S, Hess T, Kretschmar S. Radiographic detection and characteristic patterns of residual excess cement associated with cement-retained implant restorations: a clinical report. J Prosthet Dent. 2012a;107(3):151–7.

Wadhwani CP, Schuler R, Taylor S, Chen CS. Intraoral radiography and dental implant restoration. Dent Today. 2012b;31(8):66, 68, 70–1.

Wadhwani CP, Schwedhelm ER. The role of cements in dental implant success, part I. Dent Today. 2013;32(4):74–8.

White SC, Pharoah MJ. Oral radiology: principles and interpretation, Principles and interpretation. 6th ed. St. Louis: Elsevier; 2009. p. 14, 152–3.

Zwolak P, Eysel P, William-Patrick Michael J. Femoral and obturator nerves palsy caused by pelvic cement extrusion after hip arthroplasty. Orthop Rev. 2011;3(1):e6.

How Abutment Margin Design Influences Cement Flow: Abutment Selection and Cement Margin Site

6

Tomas Linkevičius

Abstract

With residual excess cement now considered a high-risk factor associated with peri-implant disease, the cement margin site needs to be scrutinized. Clinical guidance on the appropriate margin depth is always a consideration with subgingival cement margin sites, which have distinct benefits from an esthetic prospective but are higher risk for residual excess cement. In vitro as well as in vivo studies have demonstrated that this risk is reduced when equigingival and supragingival cement margins are employed. The difficulty in detecting cement clinically and with radiographs is discussed. A second in vivo study evaluates the impact of implant diameter, undercut, and implant site, evaluating the amount of cement remaining as it relates to undercut or horizontal distance between the most marginal implant neck point and the gingival margin of the restoration emergence profile. These novel, clinical-based studies help explain the complexities of implant restoration as compared with the natural tooth-cemented restoration.

Introduction

Cement-retained implant-supported restorations are a very popular way to restore dental implants. Besides many well-known advantages, this approach has drawbacks, especially the ability to adequately remove all residual excess cement (REC). Clinical research has shown that deeper subgingival cementation margins are problematic for REC despite painstaking cleaning by the clinician. Other factors, like undercut, cement properties, and location, were shown to form additional liabilities for cement removal. With the knowledge that REC is a risk factor in peri-implant disease development, abutments with cementation margins equal to or, where possible, above the free gingival margin level following the contour of conditioned peri-implant mucosa should be employed.

T. Linkevičius, DDS, Dip Pros, PhD
Department of Prosthetic Dentistry,
Institute of Odontology, Vilnius University,
Zalgiris str. 115/117, Vilnius LT 08217, Lithuania
e-mail: linktomo@gmail.com

C.P.K. Wadhwani (ed.), *Cementation in Dental Implantology: An Evidence-Based Guide*,
DOI 10.1007/978-3-642-55163-5_6, © Springer-Verlag Berlin Heidelberg 2015

Cement-Retained Restorations and Residual Excess Cement

Historically, cement-retained restorations were introduced as an esthetic solution for improperly inclined implants to avoid screw access holes, which were mandatory features of screw-retained restorations. Simple fabrication, lower costs, and similarity to tooth-borne prostheses have made this form of implant restoration the method of choice for many clinicians. Other advantages included improved passivity compared to casted screw-retained restorations, and better esthetic occlusal appearance and function, due to the absence of emergent screw access holes.

However, despite many advantages, cemented restorations have a number of shortcomings, such as predictable removal, if necessary, and inadequate retention when limited interocclusal space is present. A particular challenge now coming to light is the complete elimination of residual excess cement (REC) from the implant body, restoration, and soft peri-implant tissues. Several case reports have been published revealing complications caused by residual cement, ranging from acute severe bone resorption to implant loss. In addition, a recent study by Wilson has established a relation between residual cement and the development of chronic peri-implant disease.

One of the possible reasons for REC may be the common practice of placing implant restoration margins subgingivally. The current consensus recommends placing the cement margin of an abutment below the soft tissue level for esthetic reasons. This is done to hide the abutment-crown interface and to accommodate possible peri-implant tissue recession with time. Belser et al. recommended that the placement of the cemented margin be 1–2 mm subgingivally, which has become a common reference point for many clinicians. Furthermore, Andersson and coworkers have suggested that crown margins should be even deeper than 2 mm to achieve a better crown emergence profile. However, a recent consensus statement of the Academy of Osseointegration suggested that the threat to leave cement remnants is high when margins are deeper than 1.5 mm below tissue level. Consequently, a clinician faces the following problem: esthetic paradigms require leaving the crown margin subgingivally, which, in turn, may lead to incomplete cement cleanup and development of iatrogenic peri-implant disease. In addition, the American Academy of Periodontology recently released a report into peri-implant disease and risk factors, which, for the first time, included residual cement as a risk cause for peri-implant mucositis and peri-implantitis development. This statement brings a completely new perspective and responsibility to the restorative dentist, as cement remnant must be considered as an iatrogenic issue with serious consequences. At present, there is a lack of certainty over the depth of the margin that would not pose a threat of leaving cement undetected after cleaning.

So, how deep is safe? little has been done in implant restorative dentistry to answer this question so far. The only study to investigate this topic was performed by Agar et al. in 1997. They were the first to state that cementation of the prostheses with 1.5–3.0 mm subgingivally placed margins may lead to insufficient cement removal. Interestingly, the research itself focused more on the resulted scratching of the abutment during cleaning of cement excess, while the fact that cement remnants may not be cleaned if margins are subgingival did not receive the proper attention. Nevertheless, it still remains unclear how deep a cement margin can be placed allowing for adequate cement removal. Therefore, an initial in vitro study was undertaken, followed by clinical studies to answer this question.

The Influence of Margin Location on the Amount of Undetected Cement Excess After Delivery of Cement-Retained Restorations: In Vitro Study

Twenty-five models with embedded 3.5 mm diameter implant analogues and artificial soft gingival mask (BioHorizons, Birmingham, AL, USA) in the position of an anterior tooth were used in this study (Fig. 6.1). Individually casted abutments and the same number of metal crowns were fabricated.

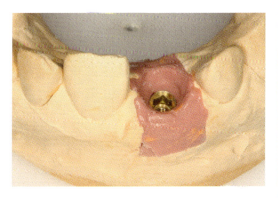

Fig. 6.1 Cast model with implant analogue and artificial soft tissue

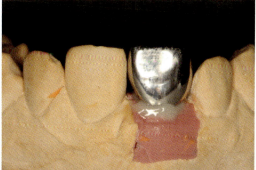

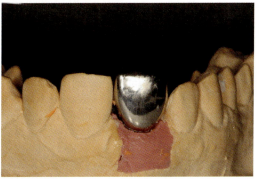

Figs. 6.3 and 6.4 Cement excess after cementation and cleaning of the crown

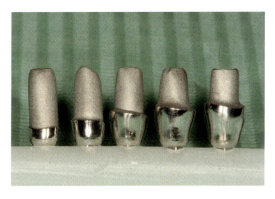

Fig. 6.2 Individually casted prosthetic abutments with different location of cementation margins

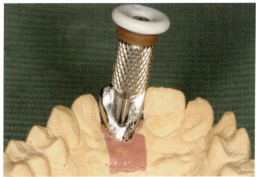

Fig. 6.5 Removal of the restoration through palatal side

Palatal openings were made in the crowns in order to have access to the abutment screw after cementation. This was necessary to ensure the retrievability of abutment/restoration system. The abutments were modeled with various positions of the margin for the restorations, consisting of five groups of five specimens (Fig. 6.2):

- Group 1 (control) at 1 mm above the gingival level
- Group 2 at the soft tissue margin
- Group 3 at 1 mm below the marginal level
- Group 4 at 2 mm below the gingival level
- Group 5 at 3 mm subgingivally

Resin-modified glass ionomer cement Fuji PLUS (GC, Tokyo, Japan) was selected as a luting agent in this study. Before cementation, the top of each prosthetic abutment was covered using dental wax to protect the abutment screw.

The palatal openings were closed with composite material to obturate the screw access space and prevent venting of luting agent during cementation. After setting, the excess was removed with a stainless steel explorer and super-floss until the researcher decided it had been completely cleaned (Figs. 6.3 and 6. 4). Then, the composite and wax were removed, the abutment screw was unscrewed, and the suprastructure was dismounted for assessment (Fig. 6.5).

Fig. 6.6 Cement remnants around abutments/crowns in different depth. Note the increase of cement as the depth of restorative margin goes deeper

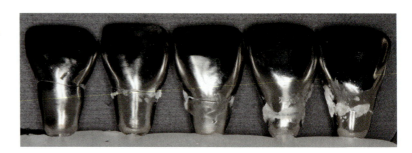

Two techniques were selected to evaluate the excess of cement left after cleaning: the computerized planimetric method of cement assessment and weighing. First, all four quadrants (mesial, distal, labial, and lingual) of the specimens were photographed using a specially constructed device to keep the standardized distance between the photo camera and the specimen. The images were imported and analyzed using Adobe Photoshop (Adobe Systems Ltd, Europe, Uxbridge, UK). Each surface area of the specimen was measured manually with the drawing facility to outline the boundaries of each quadrant. The total surface area was marked and the number of pixels was recorded from the histogram option, the same was applied to the area covered with cement remnants (Fig. 6.6). The ratio between the area covered with cement and the total surface area of the specimen was calculated. Results have shown that the increase of cement remnants in weight ($P=0.001$) and proportion ($P=0.001$) as the restoration margins were located deeper subgingivally (Kruskal–Wallis test, $P \leq 0.05$). Statistically significant differences were registered between all the groups ($P \leq 0.05$), except groups 4 and 5 ($P \geq 0.05$), when the cement excess weight was evaluated. Assessment of proportion showed statistically significant differences between all the groups ($P \leq 0.05$), except groups 1 and 2 and groups 4 and 5 ($P \geq 0.05$) (Figs. 6.7 and 6.8). Spearman's correlation coefficient showed significant relation between both measuring techniques ($r=0.889$; $P=0.001$). This means that pixel calculation is as reliable as actual weighting of the cement remnants; therefore, this method can be used also clinically.

In summary, it can be concluded that it is difficult to remove all cement excess after

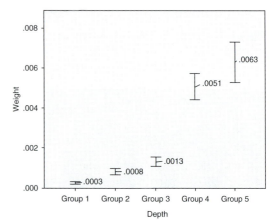

Fig. 6.7 Differences between groups in weighting

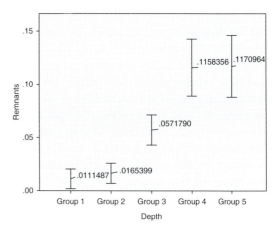

Fig. 6.8 Differences in groups in pixels

cementation if the margins are located subgingivally. The deeper the position of the margin, the greater the amount of cement can be undetected, while all cement remnants were removed only when the margin was visible. The greatest amount of cement remnants was left when the crown margin was 2 or 3 mm below the gingival level. This seems to be a logical outcome as the finish line was clearly visible and the investigator could remove the excess without difficulties. Of course, the results of laboratory study cannot be transferred directly to the clinical practice, as in vitro experiments lack essential intraoral conditions, like saliva, gingival pressure, etc. Therefore, results of in vitro study have to be tested by clinical trials if the issue is to be clinically valid.

Prospective Clinical Study

A prospective clinical study was performed to find out whether results of in vitro study could be validated by clinical trial. Sixty-five internal hexagon implants (BioHorizons Internal, Birmingham, AL, USA) were installed in 65 patients, 35 in the maxilla and 30 in the Mandibular jaw. After healing, 65 single metal-ceramic crowns with occlusal openings were fabricated. Standard prosthetic abutments were selected to support the restorations because it was important to have the same distance to cementation shoulder according to the implant. In addition, we wanted to simulate usual clinical work, as standard abutments were casually used at that time. Evaluation of the implant depth mesially, distally, lingually, and buccally was performed as the position of the cementation margin in case a standard abutment is used that varies in respect to all sites of the implant (Fig. 6.9). The data were divided into four groups according to the depth of the margin position: group 1 at the soft tissue margin, group 2 at 1 mm subgingivally, group 3 at 2 mm below marginal level, and group 4 at 3 mm subgingivally. The cementation and remnants evaluation techiques were very similar to the described preceding in vitro study. The occlusal openings of the crowns were closed with composite to prevent venting of luting agent during cementation. Resin-modified glass ionomer cement was mixed according to the manufacturer's instructions, taking the same ratio (1 little scoop of powder and 1 drop of liquid, as recommended by manufacturer) for each crown. A thin layer was applied to all the internal surfaces of

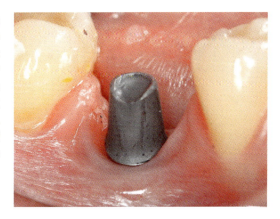

Fig. 6.9 Different depth of the cementation margin in standard abutment in respect to soft tissues

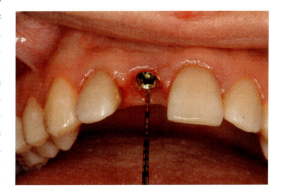

Fig. 6.10 Measurements of implant depth in four quadrants

the crowns and seated onto the abutment with a gentle finger pressure (Fig. 6.10). When setting the cement reached a rubbery consistency, the excess was removed using a stainless steel explorer, dental floss and super-floss until the researcher decided it had been completely cleaned. Then, radiographic images were made using a paralleling technique with a Rinn-like film holder in high-resolution mode. If residual cement was detected on a radiograph, cleaning procedures were repeated until a radiographic evaluation showed no cement remnants. Then the composite and wax were removed, the abutment screw was unscrewed, and the suprastructure was dismounted for assessment.

After the removal of the restoration, a photograph of the implant and surrounding tissues was made perpendicularly, using an intraoral occlusal dental mirror for evaluation of cement remnants

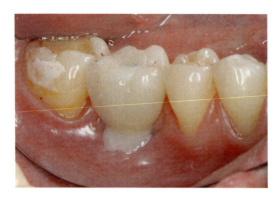

Fig. 6.11 Cementation of the restoration. Note the composite on the occlusal surface to prevent the venting of the cement

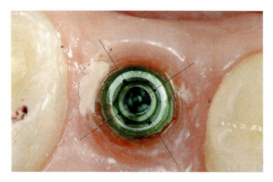

Fig. 6.12 Measurement of cement remnants in the soft peri-implant tissues after cleaning

in the tissues (Fig. 6.11). Various amounts of cement remnants were located on all retrieved superstructures and in peri-implant tissues of restored implants. Kruskal–Wallis test showed statistically significant increase of excess cement quantity on the abutment/restoration complex, as the restoration margins were located deeper subgingivally ($P=0.001$). There was a significant dependence of cement remnant amount in the peri-implant sulcus and location of the margin ($P=0.0045$). During the first radiographic evaluation, cement remnants mesially were visible in 7.5 % and in 11.3 % of all cases (Fig. 6.12).

The main finding of the study was that despite careful cleaning, various amounts of cement remnants were present on the abutment/restoration complex and in the peri-implant sulcus. The deeper the position of the margin was located, the more undetected cement particles were found

after the removal of the restoration. It is interesting to note that in all cases, when cement remnants were not cleaned, the researcher was sure that it was removed. It shows that false convictions of the clinician may contribute to the results we had. This was also registered in previous in vitro studies. Common use of standard abutments for intraoral cementation and contradicting information in the literature might be the reasons due to the misguided belief that cement removal is very easy and posses no difficulties. The properties of dental cement may also have had influence on the results of this clinical trial. Almost two decades ago, Agar et al. showed that dental cement containing resins was the most difficult to remove from the surface of abutments. In addition, the removal of such cement resulted in the most extensive scratching of the metal surface.

Likewise, a recent survey has shown that glass ionomer modified with resins is the most popular cement to use for permanent delivery of implant-supported restorations in US dental schools, reaching up to 70 % of usage. This clinical study could suggest the recommendation that clinicians should select cement with less adhesive characteristics for cementation of implant restorations, like zinc phosphate, whose cleaning properties are much superior to other cements. One of the factors to explain this phenomenon probably lies in the process of conventional cementing restorations on teeth. During seating, hydraulic pressure builds up and cement travels to the direction of least resistance, through the margin to the gingival sulcus. However, the perpendicular fiber attachment around teeth provides a sufficient barrier, and cement excess does not penetrate further and escapes to the surface of the gingival sulcus, where it is more readily detected. It is well known that peri-implant tissues do not possess similar protective mechanisms and are less resistant to pressure. Thus, cement excess may be pushed further subgingivally with only a part of it escaping to the surface. In contrast to teeth, the peri-implant tissues lack resistance to pressure due to the absence of an attachment to the implant surface. Connective tissue fibers do not attach to the implant and align themselves parallel along the fixture surface. Subsequently, the peri-implant tissues may be less resistant to pressure compared with tissues around teeth. Several studies have shown that pressure ranging from 20 to 130 N can be developed during the cementation of crowns. This would suggest that cement may be pushed deeper in the peri-implant sulcus and defy removal even after meticulous attempts at cleaning.

Validity of Radiographic Evaluation

The most interesting finding was that radiographic examination could not be trusted to detect pieces of cement. It is obvious that it is impossible to inspect the palatine/lingual and facial areas due to the obstruction of the implant/abutment complex. Traditionally, proximal areas are considered the mostly likely place where cement extrusion can be easily detected, although usually the soft tissues are thicker here due to the presence of papillae. However, results of this clinical study have shown that this is not necessarily the case. Cement remnants were visible medially only in two cases and in five cases distally out of 35 radiographic images, 5.7 and 14.3 %, respectively. A partial explanation to that may be found in the study by Wadhwani et al., which has proved that radiographic density of implant restorative cements is rather poor and greatly depends on the thickness of the specimens. For example, resin-reinforced glass ionomer used in this study could be detected only when cement thickness of 2 mm was irradiated. This means that smaller particles of excess cement are not visible even proximally, where no blocking of the implant body exists. In addition, very frequently, however, because the cement tends to flow circumferentially around implant restorations, there are occasions when even thin layers can be detected radiographically. Provided the clinician understands this phenomenon, known as the peripheral egg shell effect (see chapter 5). This increases the observed radiographic effect as the thin circumferetial layer attenuates the x-ray beam at a tangent-making it more likley to be seen (Fig. 6.13a–e). Wadhwani et al. have described

a few additional situations when radiographic examination was not able to detect cement remnants, such as in cement superimposition, when cement is on a metallic surface and is almost impossible to detect. Other situations may arise when radiolucent cement is used. Within the limitations of the study, the following conclusions could be drawn:

1. The deeper the position of the margin, the more undetected cement could be found after cleaning adhered to abutment/restoration complex and in per-implant tissues. Abutments with visible margins could be recommended for intraoral cementation.
2. Radiographic examination should only be a supplementary method for detection of cement excess.
3. The use of standard abutments for cementation with permanent cement should be very careful or completely suspended due to the high risk of cement excess.

Undercut, Implant Position, and Diameter

There are several other factors besides the depth of the cementation margin which may influence the amount of cement remnants. The role of clinical factors such as location of the implant (anterior or posterior), implant diameter, and the effect of an undercut around the implant is still not known. The first important parameter that should be discussed is the undercut or negative angle (Fig. 6.14a, b).

According to "The Glossary of Prosthodontic Terms," undercut is defined as an angle formed by any surface of the tooth below the survey line of the height of contour, with the selected path of insertion of prosthesis. In the implant dentistry cement-related topic, undercut could be defined as a difference between cementation (cement extrusion line) line and the line of exit of the restoration emergence profile from peri-implant tissues. In this study, the undercut definition was specified to be the distance from the most marginal implant neck point (line B, C, F, G) to the gingival margin of the restoration's emergence

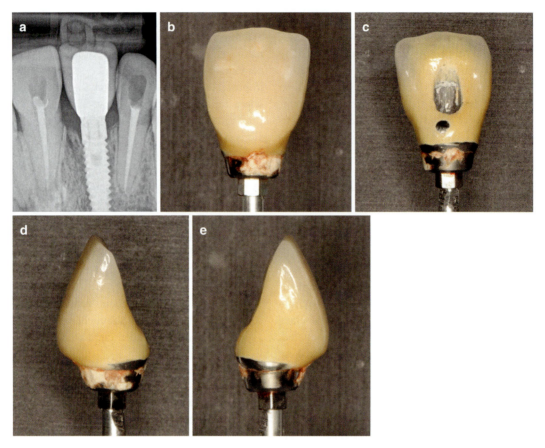

Fig. 6.13 (**a**) X-ray of the implant crown, no cement remnants are visible; (**b**) the same retrieved abutment/restoration with visible cement remnants buccally, (**c**) lingually, and (**d, e**) interproximally

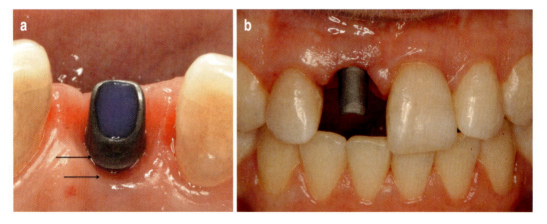

Fig. 6.14 (**a, b**) Undercut of the standard abutment. Cementation line (*upper arrow*) and the restoration emergence profile line (*lower arrow*)

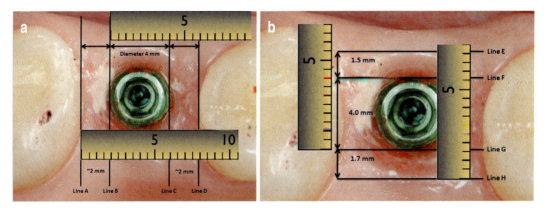

Fig. 6.15 (**a**, **b**) Measurement of mesiodistal and buccolingual undercuts

profile (line E, H) or to the adjacent teeth (line D, A) in the horizontal plane (Fig. 6.15a, b).

This undercut was measured in four locations: Distance from the most marginal implant's neck point to the adjacent tooth mesially and distally (distance between lines: from A to B and from C to D) and distance from the most marginal implant neck point to the outer margin of the soft tissues buccally and lingually (distance between lines: from E to F and from G to H).

The data (65 single crowns with 4 measurements = 260 samples) was divided into three groups according to the extent of the undercut:

- Group 1 (118 samples): up to 1 mm
- Group 2 (96 samples): from 1 to 2 mm
- Group 3 (46 samples): 3 mm and more

Results have shown that there was a strong relationship between the undercut and residual cement in the soft tissues ($P=0.004$) and on the crown/abutment complex ($P=0.046$). Mann–Whitney test showed the statistically significant increase of the undetected cement in both groups when the undercut became greater from 1 to 2 mm (soft tissue $P=0.002$ and crown/abutment P 0.005)

Surprisingly, no studies analyzed the impact of the undercuts' influence on the cement removal. Nevertheless, it seems that the impact of the latter factor is obvious. Study data shows that greater undercut results in more undetected cement being left after cleaning. Even though the

amount of cement remnants increased when the undercut became greater, the statistical significance had been detected only between 1 and 2 mm in both groups (on the abutment and in the soft tissues). This proves that the usage of the standard abutments to support cement-retained implant restorations must be strictly avoided, because the shoulder of the standard abutment does not follow the line of the gingiva and emergence profile of the implant. It is important to note that a lot of cement remains undetected when the undercut is extensive, even though the cementation margin is not very deep (Fig. 6.16a, b).

Another interesting factor is implant diameter. Implant diameter is correlated with restorative abutment diameter, which is closely related to the extent of the undercut. We have evaluated 65 internal hex implants (BioHorizons Internal, Birmingham, AL, USA), consisting of 21 implants of 3.5 mm (32.3 %), 34 implants of 4.0 mm (52.3 %), and 10 implants of 5.0 mm (15.4 %) diameter. The results have shown statistically significant decrease of the remaining cement in the soft tissues when implant diameter got wider ($P=0.026$); however, there was no significant relationship found concerning cement left on the abutment and diameter ($P=0.600$). The Mann–Whitney test compared the groups separately, and statistically significant difference was found in the soft tissue group between 4.0 and 5.0 mm diameters ($P=0.009$). Location of

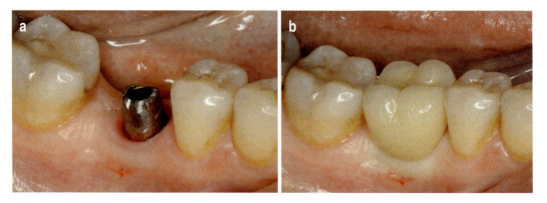

Fig. 6.16 (**a**, **b**) Cementation margin is not deep; however, mesiodistal undercut is extensive; therefore, cement remnants would not be removed in this case

the implant (anterior, premolar, and molar) did not have any influence of cement excess amount.

Conclusion

Several clinical recommendations could be suggested according to the results of our laboratory and clinical studies. First, standard abutment should not be used for intraoral cementation with permanent cement due to the issues discussed in this chapter. Cementation margin position and extent of undercut seem to be the most important factors, which influence the amount of cement remnants in peri-implant tissues and/or abutment/restoration.

Further, individual, or custom abutments with supragingival or epigingival margins, following the contour of the peri-implant tissues, should be used to support the implant restoration intraorally. Individual abutments not only allow raising the cementation margin to the level where cement can be safely cleaned, they also eliminate the undercut as well, because cementation margin coincides with emergence profile of the restoration.

Further more, peri-implant soft tissues are supported by the abutment material, not the crown suprastructure and usually covered with ceramics. As highly biocompatible materials like titanium and zirconium are available for fabrication of patient-specific abutments, peri-implant soft tissues may greatly benefit from this use of individual approach. The use of indi-

vidual abutments reduces the importance of radiographic examination, because the clinician can see the cement extrusion site and thus can remove the excess. It is obvious that margin visibility plays a crucial role in cement elimination. This can be compared with the study by Christensen, who tested marginal fit of gold inlay castings with visible and not visible clinical examination margins. It was concluded that an explorer examination of visually accessible gold inlay margins is superior to and more reliable than an explorer or radiographic examination of visually inaccessible margins.

Finally, a screw-retained approach also could be considered if cement remnants present a problem that needs to be completely eliminated.

Bibliography

Academy of Prosthodontics. The glossary of prosthodontic terms. J Prosthet Dent. 2005;94:10–92.

Agar JR, Cameron SM, Hughbanks JC, Parker MH. Cement removal from restorations luted to titanium abutments with simulated subgingival margins. J Prosthet Dent. 1997;78:43–7.

Andersson B, Odman P, Lindvall AM, Branemark PI. Cemented single crowns on osseointegrated implants after 5 years: results from a prospective study on CeraOne. Int J Prosthodont. 1998;11:212–8.

Belser UC, Buser D, Hess D, Schmid B, Bernard JP, Lang NP. Aesthetic implant restorations in partially edentulous patients – a critical appraisal. Periodontol 2000. 1998;17:132–50.

Belser U, Buser D, Higginbottom F. Consensus statements and recommended clinical procedures regarding esthetics in implant dentistry. Int J Oral Maxillofac Implants. 2004;19(Suppl):73–4.

Berglundh T, Lindhe J, Marinello C, Ericsson I, Liljenberg B. Soft tissue reaction to de novo plaque formation on implants and teeth. An experimental study in the dog. Clin Oral Implants Res. 1992;3:1–8.

Blatz MB, Bergler M, Holst S, Block MS. Zirconia abutments for single-tooth implants – rationale and clinical guidelines. J Oral Maxillofac Surg. 2009;67(11 Suppl):74–81.

Caudry S, Chvartszaid D, Kemp N. A simple cementation method to prevent material extrusion into the periimplant tissues. J Prosthet Dent. 2009;102:130–1.

Chee W, Felton DA, Johnson PF, Sullivan DY. Cemented versus screw-retained implant prostheses: which is better? Int J Oral Maxillofac Implants. 1999;14: 137–41.

Cheshire PD, Hobkirk JA. An in vivo quantitative analysis of the fit of Nobel Biocare implant superstructures. J Oral Rehabil. 1996;23:782–9.

Cochran DL, Hermann JS, Schenk RK, Higginbottom FL, Buser D. Biologic width around titanium implants. A histometric analysis of the implanto-gingival junction around unloaded and loaded non-submerged implants in the canine mandible. J Periodontol. 1997;68: 186–98.

Cohen RB, Hallmon WW, Culliton CR, Herbold ET. Bacteriostatic effect of tetracycline in a temporary cement. J Prosthet Dent. 1989;62:607–9.

Ericsson I, Lindhe J. Probing depth at implants and teeth. An experimental study in the dog. J Clin Periodontol. 1993;20:623–7.

Gapski R, Neugeboren N, Pomeranz AZ, Reissner MW. Endosseous implant failure influenced by crown cementation: a clinical case report. Int J Oral Maxillofac Implants. 2008;23:943–6.

No authors listed. Glossary of prosthodontic terms. J Prosthet Dent 2005;94:10–92.

Hebel KS, Gajjar RC. Cement-retained versus screw-retained implant restorations: achieving optimal occlusion and esthetics in implant dentistry. J Prosthet Dent. 1997;77:28–35.

Higginbottom F, Belser U, Jones JD, Keith SE. Prosthetic management of implants in the esthetic zone. Int J Oral Maxillofac Implants. 2004;19(Suppl):62–72.

Jung RE, Pjetursson BE, Glauser R, Zembic A, Zwahlen M, Lang NP. A systematic review of the 5-year survival and complication rates of implant-supported single crowns. Clin Oral Implants Res. 2008;19:119–30.

Jung RE, Zembic A, Pjetursson BE, Zwahlen M, Thoma DS. Systematic review of the survival rate and the incidence of biological, technical and esthetic complications of single crowns on implants reported in longitudinal studies with a mean follow-up of 5 years. Clin Oral Implants Res. 2012;23 Suppl 6:2–21.

Korsch M, Obst U, Walther W. Cement-associated peri-implantitis: a retrospective clinical observational study of fixed implant-supported restorations using a meth-

acrylate cement. Clin Oral Implants Res. 2014;25: 797–802.

Lee A, Okayasu K, Wang HL. Screw- versus cement-retained implant restorations: current concepts. Implant Dent. 2010;19:8–15.

Lewis S, Avera S, Engleman M, Beumer J. The restoration of improperly inclined osseointegrated implants. Int J Oral Maxillofac Implants. 1989;4:147–52.

Lewis S, Beumer III J, Hornburg W, Moy P. The "UCLA" abutment. Int J Oral Maxillofac Implants. 1988;3:183–9.

Lindhe J, Berglundh T, Ericsson I, Liljenberg B, Marinello C. Experimental breakdown of peri-implant and periodontal tissues. A study in the beagle dog. Clin Oral Implants Res. 1992;3:9–16.

Linkevicius T, Vindasiute E, Puisys A, Peciuliene V. The influence of margin location on the amount of undetected cement excess after delivery of cement-retained implant restorations. Clin Oral Implants Res. 2011a;22:1379–84.

Linkevicius T, Vindasiute E, Puisys A, Linkeviciene L, Maslova N, Puriene A. The influence of the cementation margin position on the amount of undetected cement. A prospective clinical study. Clin Oral Implants Res. 2013a;24:71–6.

Linkevicius T, Svediene O, Vindasiute E, Linkeviciene L. A technique for making impressions of deeply placed implants. J Prosthet Dent. 2011b;106:204–5.

Linkevicius T, Puisys A, Vindasiute E, Linkeviciene L, Apse P. Does residual cement around implant-supported restorations cause peri-implant disease? A retrospective case analysis. Clin Oral Implants Res. 2013b;24:1179–84.

Michalakis KX, Hirayama H, Garefis PD. Cement-retained versus screw-retained implant restorations: a critical review. Int J Oral Maxillofac Implants. 2003;18:719–28.

Moráguez OD, Belser UC. The use of polytetrafluoroethylene tape for the management of screw access channels in implant-supported prostheses. J Prosthet Dent. 2010;103:189–91.

Nissan J, Narobai D, Gross O, Ghelfan O, Chaushu G. Long-term outcome of cemented versus screw-retained implant-supported partial restorations. Int J Oral Maxillofac Implants. 2011;26:1102–7.

Patel D, Invest JC, Tredwin CJ, Setchell DJ, Moles DR. An analysis of the effect of a vent hole on excess cement expressed at the crown- abutment margin for cement-retained implant crowns. J Prosthodont. 2009;18:54–9.

Pauletto N, Lahiffe BJ, Walton JN. Complications associated with excess cement around crowns on osseointegrated implants: a clinical report. Int J Oral Maxillofac Implants. 1999;14:865–8.

Preiskel HW, Tsolka P. Telescopic prostheses for implants. Int J Oral Maxillofac Implants. 1998;13:352–7.

Rajan M, Gunaseelan R. Fabrication of a cement- and screw-retained implant prosthesis. J Prosthet Dent. 2004;92:578–80.

Sailer I, Zembic A, Jung RE, Siegenthaler D, Holderegger C, Hämmerle CH. Randomized controlled clinical trial of customized zirconia and titanium implant abutments for canine and posterior single-tooth implant reconstructions: preliminary results at 1 year of function. Clin Oral Implants Res. 2009;20: 219–25.

Shor A, Schuler R, Goto Y. Indirect implant-supported fixed provisional restoration in the esthetic zone: fabrication technique and treatment workflow. J Esthet Restor Dent. 2008;20:82–95.

Tarica DY, Alvarado VM, Truong ST. Survey of United States dental schools on cementation protocols for implant crown restorations. J Prosthet Dent. 2010;103:68–79.

Taylor TD, Agar JR. Twenty years of progress in implant prosthodontics. J Prosthet Dent. 2002;88:89–95.

Vigolo P, Givani A, Majzoub Z, Cordioli G. Cemented versus screw-retained implant-supported single-tooth crowns: a 4-year prospective clinical study. Int J Oral Maxillofac Implants. 2004;19:260–5.

Wadhwani C, Hess T, Faber T, Piñeyro A, Chen CSK. A descriptive study of the radiographic density of implant restorative cements. J Prosthet Dent. 2010;103:295–302.

White DJ. Dental calculus: recent insights into occurrence, formation, prevention, removal and oral health effects of supragingival and subgingival deposits. Eur J Oral Sci. 1997;105:508–22.

Wilson Jr TG. The positive relationship between excess cement and peri-implant disease: a prospective clinical endoscopic study. J Periodontol. 2009;80: 1388–92.

Restorative Options That Eliminate or Reduce the Potential for Cement-Induced Peri-implant Disease

7

Chandur P.K. Wadhwani and Tomas Linkevičius

Abstract

With the knowledge that cement-retained restorative options for treating implant sites may increase the risk for disease, screw-retained solutions are being considered. Dealing with the screw access channel esthetics and ability to control occlusal force has been considered the primary motivation for the use of cement-retained implant restorations. The implant crown with an esthetic plug was published to offer a solution to this problem. Using currently available materials, any dental laboratory capable of pressing ceramic porcelains can use this design and improve both the esthetics and occlusal contacting site. The cement-screw restoration is described as another alternative. This takes advantage of extraoral cementation of the restoration onto the abutment, which negates the problem of pushing cement down into the vulnerable soft tissues, and then using the screw(s) to lock the crown or bridge to the implant body.

Where esthetic demands are high and the screw channel angulation an issue, using supragingival margins that allow for ceramic to ceramic bonding is described in the implant crown with an esthetic adhesive margin section. This design uses porcelains that are bonded and matched producing a highly effective result.

Implant companies are also developing new abutment designs to further promote the use of screw-retained restorations. Using novel screwdrivers and funneling the screw around angle changes appear to be a promising solution for the future.

C.P.K. Wadhwani, BDS (Hons), MSD (✉)
Department of Restorative Dentistry, University of Washington School of Dentistry, Seattle, WA, USA

Private Practice Limited to Prosthodontics, 1200, 116th Ave NE #A, Bellevue, WA 98004, USA
e-mail: cpkw@uw.edu

T. Linkevičius, DDS, Dip Pros, PhD
Department of Prosthetic Dentistry, Institute of Odontology, Vilnius University, Zalgiris str. 115/117, Vilnius LT 08217, Lithuania
e-mail: linktomo@gmail.com

C.P.K. Wadhwani (ed.), *Cementation in Dental Implantology: An Evidence-Based Guide*,
DOI 10.1007/978-3-642-55163-5_7, © Springer-Verlag Berlin Heidelberg 2015

Introduction

This chapter will focus on restorative options that either eliminate the possibility of cement extrusion into the peri-implant tissues—for example, by using an implant-screw-retained option—or by means of gaining complete control of the cement margin site during the cementation procedure.

Using Screw-Retained Restorative Options for Implant Restorations

Screw-retained implant crowns may be clinically demanding, especially managing the esthetic and occlusal challenges of screw access channel closure. Many clinicians have moved away from using screw retention as a means of fixing a crown to an implant in favor of cementation to an underlying abutment. This has occurred primarily in response to esthetic challenges and because cementation is routinely used in conventional tooth form dentistry, so dentists appear to be familiar with the materials and processes. However, a link has been established between peri-implant disease and excess cement extrusion in cement-retained implant restorations. This chapter describes a novel technique of bonding a pressed porcelain plug into the screw access channel of an implant restoration, which allows for control of occlusion, matches the esthetics of a cement-retained crown, and eliminates the issues of excess cement.

From the 1980s to early 1990s, implant prostheses were primarily screw retained. This preference changed with the introduction of components that allowed for cement retention of implant restorations. Factors that have contributed to the rise in popularity of the cementation procedures include esthetics, control of occlusion, less demanding implant placement, cost (component and laboratory), improved passive fit for multiple connected units, and similarity to conventional tooth-supported fixed prosthodontics.

Cement-retained restorations, however, are not without their issues. It has been reported that when comparing screw-retained implant restorations with cemented implant restorations,

a measurable difference in health (modified plaque index, bleeding index) was noted, with the cement-retained crowns worsening over time. Sinus tracts, inflammation, and continued bone loss have been documented as being related to cement residue remaining in the peri-implant soft tissues. A recent study reported on the positive relationship between excess cement and peri-implant disease (peri-mucositis and peri-implantitis). These conditions are classified as inflammatory lesions which may affect the peri-implant tissues, with the potential loss of supporting bone. Although it is possible to treat peri-implant disease, prevention is the goal of supportive therapy. Techniques have been developed to minimize the extrusion of luting cement into the peri-implant soft tissues, but it is likely that these issues cannot be predictably eliminated. The inability to completely remove cement from the implant-abutment surfaces and the difficulties in radiographic detection of some commonly used luting cements have been reported.

It would seem better to avoid these problems entirely by using a screw-retained restoration; however, this requires closure of the screw access channel, which most commonly is achieved with a direct restoration that may compromise esthetics. It has been reported that the screw hole can occupy up to 50 % of the occlusal table, and when the screw hole is located directly over the implant, vertical loading is difficult, which may compromise biomechanics.

Screw access closure is frequently considered a provisional procedure due to screw loosening, with little attention given to the restorative material. However, recent systemic reviews suggest that abutment screw loosening is a rare event in single-implant restorations. This is regardless of the geometry of implant-abutment connection and provided that the proper anti-rotational features and torque are employed.

The Screw-Retained Implant Crown with an Adhesive Plug (ICAP)

A clinical report documented the use of a screw-retained custom metal-ceramic abutment combined with an adhesively bonded porcelain restoration as a permanent solution to an implant inclination issue combined with a short clinical crown. Traditional porcelain stacking processes produced equigingival and supragingival margins on an abutment to which a porcelain suprastructure was adhesively bonded—a type III veneer. While this technique is innovative, it is time consuming and requires the dental laboratory technician be highly skilled. Use of a pressed porcelain system that requires only moderate laboratory time and less demanding technical skills is described. The implant crown adhesive plug (ICAP) consists of a pressed metal-ceramic screw-retained crown with the access channel closed by a custom-pressed porcelain plug that is shaped and shade matched to the crown. The pressed ceramic plug is etched, silanated, and adhesively bonded with composite lute into the crown—similar to an inlay. This type of restoration eliminates some of the disadvantages associated with screw-retained crowns, such as the unesthetic appearance of the screw channel and disruption of the occlusal contact area. It also eliminates cement contact with the peri-implant tissues which could be negatively affected by chemicals within the cement.

Clinical Report: Case 1

A 60-year-old female patient required restoration of both premolar and molar dental implants (Replace Select, Nobel Biocare USA, Yorba Linda, CA, USA). The implants were optimally placed using a surgical guide designed and fabricated according to the patient's restorative needs. After fixing the appropriate impression copings to the implants, an open-tray implant-level impression was made in vinyl polysiloxane (Aquasil Ultra, Dentsply, York, PA, USA). In the laboratory, analogs (Nobel Biocare) were attached to the impression copings (Nobel Biocare), and an implant cast fabricated that incorporated a soft tissue gingival mask (Gingitech, Ivoclar Vivadent, Schaan, Liechtenstein) with a type IV stone (Fujirock, GC, Leuven, Belgium).

Cast-to laboratory abutments (Nobel Biocare) were fixed to the implant analogs and waxed to full contour from which a putty matrix (Sil-Tech, Ivoclar Vivadent, Schaan, Liechtenstein) was made. The matrix provided a cutback guide for the metal framework dimensions needed to support porcelain. The wax pattern incorporating the cast-to abutment was sprued, invested (Microstar HS Investment, Microstar Dental, Lawrenceville, GA, USA), and casted in porcelain bonding alloy (JP1, Jensen Industries, North Haven, CT, USA) according to the manufacturer's instructions. The casting, once divested and cleaned, was opaqued (Pulse Opaque, Ceramay, Stuttgart, Germany) with the required shade and sintered.

The putty index was used to make a full contour waxing over the opaqued framework. A cast custom metal key was warmed and inserted into the screw access channel through the wax up (Fig. 7.1a, b).

Wax replicas of the key (Geo, Renfert, Hilzingen, Germany) were produced by placing the shank of the key in a putty matrix for a mold, then injecting with molten wax. The wax key replica was inserted and contoured (Fig. 7.2a, b) to form the wax plug.

The contoured wax plug and crown were attached to the same sprue (Fig. 7.3a) and invested in porcelain pressing investment (Microstar HS Investment, Microstar Dental, Lawrenceville, GA, USA). The appropriate shade of ingot was selected (Pulse Press-To-Metal ingot, Jensen Industries, New Haven, CT, USA), and the pressing was made following the manufacturer's recommendations in the pressing furnace (Vario Press 300, Zubler, Ulm, Germany). The pressed ceramic was recovered using airborne particle abrasion with the engaging surfaces of the implant crown protected with a layer of wax (Fig. 7.3b).

The porcelain plug was opaqued on the internal aspect to prevent gray show-through of the metal screw channel. The porcelain of the crown and plug was customized with stains and glazed.

The fitting surfaces of the porcelain were prepared for adhesive bonding by etching with 9 % hydrofluoric acid (Porcelain Etch, Ultradent Products Inc., South Jordan, UT, USA) for 90 s, then rinsed for 20 s. Further cleaning with 35 % phosphoric acid (Ultra-Etch, Ultradent Products Inc., South Jordan, UT, USA) for 30 s and a 20-s rinse followed. Finally, cleaning was completed by separate immersion of the crown and plug in distilled water in an ultrasonic bath for 5 min.

Fig. 7.1 (**a**) Custom occlusal metal key forms occlusal screw access channel with wax replica of screw channel pattern. (**b**) Custom metal key placed in the premolar waxing, forming occlusal screw access channel pattern seen in molar

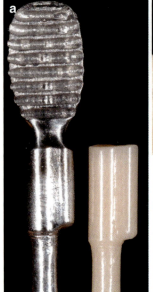
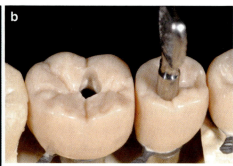

Fig. 7.2 (**a**) Wax replica key pattern placed in the premolar screw access channel. (**b**) Wax key pattern shaped to conform to the occlusal morphology of the premolar

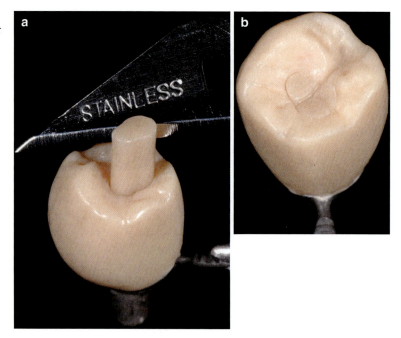

The bonding surfaces were silanated (Silane, Ultradent Products Inc., South Jordan, UT, USA) following thorough oil-free air drying and dried at 100 °C for 5 min in the oven.

To avoid saliva contamination of the fitting surfaces of the abutment crown, rubber dam isolation was used. After radiographic confirmation of complete seating, the screw was tightened to the appropriate torque (35 Ncm). A small pellet of sterilized polytetrafluoroethylene (PTFE) tape (Oatey Co, Cleveland, OH, USA) was placed over the screwhead, and the previously etched

Fig. 7.3 (**a**) Wax crown and plug simultaneously sprued and ready to invest for pressing in porcelain. (**b**) Pressed crown and plug in porcelain (a layer of blue wax protects the implant-abutment interfacing surfaces during airborne particle abrasion)

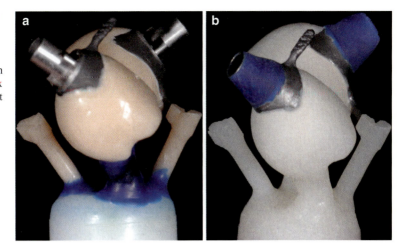

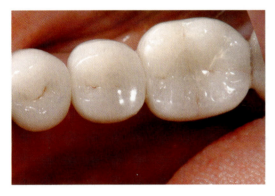

Fig. 7.4 Clinical view ICAP of the molar and premolar case shown after seating and bonding in the pressed porcelain plug

and silanated porcelain surfaces were then coated with adhesive resin (Prime and Bond, Dentsply, York, PA, USA) followed by the application of resin luting agent (Ultra Bond Plus, DenMat, Santa Maria, CA, USA). The plug was seated and held in place for light polymerization. The final ICAP was cleaned of excess resin, occlusion evaluated and adjusted, and the crown polished with porcelain polishing points; the results of which are shown in Fig. 7.4 (Dialite, Brasseler USA, Savannah, GA, USA).

Clinical Report: Case 2

A 64-year-old female presented with an osseointegrated implant in the lower left first premolar region. The implant (Endopore, Sybron, Orange, CA, USA) was previously restored with a

cement-retained single crown that was causing some soft tissue irritation as a result of excess cement extrusion into the peri-implant tissues (Fig. 7.5a). Due to the lingual inclination of the implant, traditional filling of the screw access channel would result in an unsightly and difficult restoration. The ICAP was used to overcome these issues. The crown's metal substructure was casted and opaque applied. A full contour waxing was made (Fig. 7.5b), and in this instance due to the complexity of the case, the pressed ceramic porcelain fused to metal crown was fabricated prior to the ceramic plug.

Once fabricated, the internal aspect of the ceramic plug was opaqued (Fig. 7.6a, b), and the bonding surfaces were etched and silanated to allow for adhesive resin bonding as described earlier (Fig. 7.7a, b). The crown was delivered and screwed to the appropriate torque, with rubber dam placed for isolation and the porcelain plug cemented.

The ICAP is a restoration that has three major advantages, which include improved esthetics, controlled occlusion, and the elimination of potential cement-induced peri-implant disease. It is a durable, esthetic restoration that can be economically made with moderate skills in the dental laboratory. This type of restoration can also be used for fixed bridges, with the inlay providing both an esthetic and occlusal contact advantage over simply filling of the occlusal screw access with materials such as composite resin.

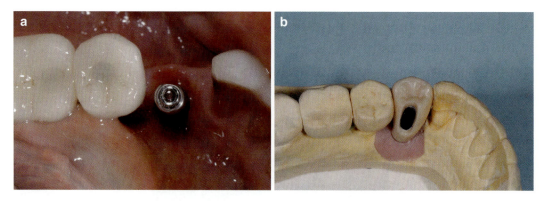

Fig. 7.5 (**a**) Implant position. Note lingual inclination. (**b**) Full contour waxing prior to pressing in porcelain (metal framework within and screw access shown)

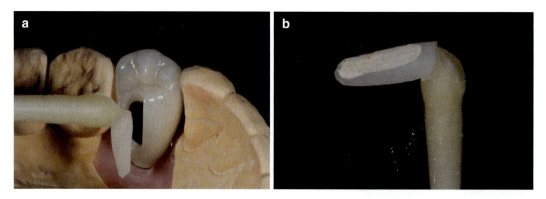

Fig. 7.6 (**a**) Pressed ceramic crown with pressed porcelain screw access channel plug. (**b**) Porcelain pressed porcelain plug; note opaque on intaglio surface of plug to prevent metal show-through

The Cement-Screw Restoration

The recent introduction of the cement-screw-retained restoration has been described, which combines some features from both the cement- and screw-retained restorations. The system consists of the crown with occlusal opening, which is cemented on prepared standard abutment or special retentive metal base on the working model. The cement excess is cleaned and restoration is screwed to the implant in the mouth. This approach assures passive fit of the restoration, as cement layer is present between crown and abutment. Consequently, occlusal opening for connection to the implant makes it similar to screw-retained restoration. This technique is very cost effective and can be used for single crowns and for short-span fixed partial dentures as well.

When the time to restore implants arrives, traditionally clinicians can choose between cemented or screw-retained restorations. We all know the advantages of the cemented approach—passive fit, esthetic, and functional occlusal surface; in short, the possibility to solve the problems with poorly positioned implants. However, the main disadvantage of cemented restorations is of course possible cement extrusion into peri-implant tissues and difficulties in removing the remnants. Problems also arise if the cemented crown becomes mobile due to abutment screw loosening, as then occlusal perforation must be made to reach the screw and tighten it back.

The other option which may be chosen is to use screw-retained restorations. It is a cement-free solution, free from remnant-associated complications. However, casting technology frequently

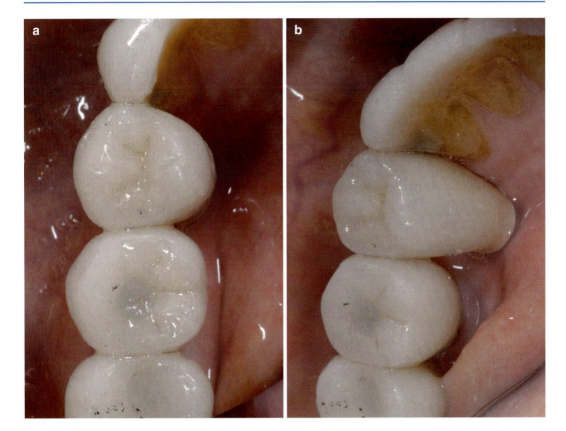

Fig. 7.7 (**a**, **b**) Clinical views of the ICAP—occlusal and lingual of lower left first premolar with lingual plug

resulted in screw loosening, fractures, and veneering porcelain fractures in the past. These complications frequently restrained clinicians from using screw-retained restorations.

Current dental technologies allow solving major problems of cemented and screw-retained restorations. It is simply to use individual abutments with margins following contours of peri-implant tissues, which will certainly reduce cement excess-related complications. Screw-retained frameworks can be milled, thus eliminating inner tension problems inherited from casting. However, these improvements come with a price—individual abutments and milling costs usually are much higher than the cost of standard solutions.

As a possible solution, a cement-screw-retained restoration is described. It consists of the crown with occlusal opening, which is cemented on a prepared standard abutment on the working model. Cement excess is cleaned, and restoration is screwed to the implant in the mouth. This construction eliminates the cement remnants, as the crown is glued to the abutment on the model and the technician can easily remove cement excess. Biomechanically this kind of restoration is cement retained; thus, passive fit is achieved due to the layer of the cement between the abutment and the crown. The use of standard abutments eliminates the need to make expensive framework milling.

Different bases can be used for retention of cement-screw-retained restorations. If the implant needs to be restored with single restoration, the clinician can choose from standard stock abutment or specially designed titanium base. If fixed partial denture is to be constructed, non-hexed titanium bases could be used for retention of the supra-structure.

This technique allows using metal-ceramic and zirconium-ceramic restorations as well. Only slight difference in metallic base treatment and cementation agent should be noticed.

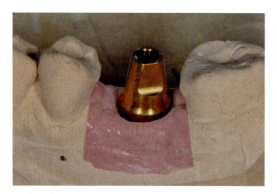

Fig. 7.8 Standard abutment

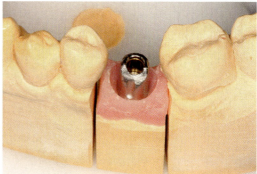

Fig. 7.9 Prepared abutment with deep cementation margins

Rajan and Gunaseelan described a very similar technique of cement-screw-retained restoration. They also proposed to use standard abutments and metal-ceramic restoration with occlusal opening; however, the cementation procedure was to be performed intraorally. After that, abutment-restoration complex was retrieved, cement remnants cleaned, and the restoration returned to the mouth.

Our proposed technique has several advantages. First, the cementation procedure is more controlled on the model than in the mouth, especially if the implant is placed deeply. In such a case, it is difficult to seat the crown on implant in the mouth, due to resistance of the peri-implant tissues. Secondly, less clinical time is spent, as cementation and excess cleaning procedures are done in the laboratory.

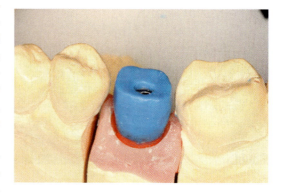

Fig. 7.10 Waxing of the metal framework of the cement-screw-retained restoration

Standard Abutment

The fabrication of single cement-screw-retained implant restoration with standard abutment as a base starts with positioning the abutment in the model (Fig. 7.8). Then it is prepared for restoration. As cementation of the crown will be performed on the model, the cementation margin can be positioned at the deepest point, in this way increasing all the surface of the abutment and increasing retention of the crown (Fig. 7.9). Then the framework is waxed and casted from metal with occlusal opening for the screw (Figs. 7.10 and 7.11). The framework is veneered with ceramics and is not attached to the abutment yet (Fig. 7.12a, b). The final laboratory stage includes

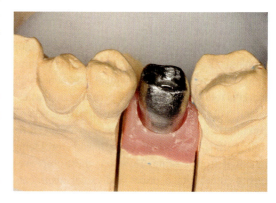

Fig. 7.11 Metal framework with occlusal hole

the cementation of the finished and glazed metal-ceramic restoration on the abutment (Fig. 7.13 and Fig. 7.14). After cement excess removal and polishing, the cement-screw-retained restoration is

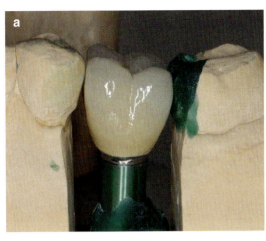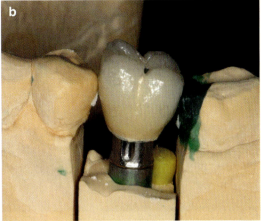

Fig. 7.12 (**a**, **b**) Ceramics are applied on metal framework

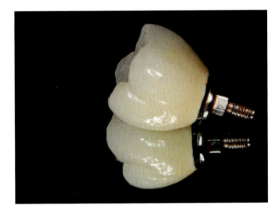

Fig. 7.13 Glazed crown is cemented on standard abutment, and cement excess is cleaned

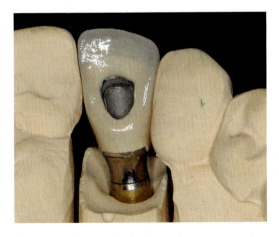

Fig. 7.14 The completed Cemented-Screw restoration. Note: The abutment is visible within the screw access hole

screwed to the implant (Fig. 7.14). The access hole is etched with hydrofluoric acid, primed, and covered with composite (Fig. 7.15a, b). The control radiographic image shows precise seating of the restoration on the integrated implant (Fig. 7.16).

Titanium Base

Titanium base also could be used for fabrication of single cement-screw-retained restoration, when more esthetics and biocompatibility is required. In fact, these titanium bases are more designed to use zirconium-based crowns, as usually they are a bit shorter and have "metal-free window," which is designed to reduce the shine-through of the base metal through zirconium. However, if an implant is placed deep, the base is buried under the tissues, and this becomes not so important. The sequence of the clinical and laboratory steps is similar to previously described.

In the clinical situation described, two implants (BioHorizons Tapered, Birmingham, AL, USA) are placed in the first and second mandibular molar tooth sites. Soft peri-implant tissues have been conditioned with temporary screw-retained restorations and are ready for prosthetic rehabilitation (Fig. 7.17a). Titanium bases are selected for a support of zirconium-ceramic restoration (Fig. 7.17b). An open impression is taken to register implant position and peri-implant soft tissue contour.

First the wax replica of the future zirconium framework is created by the technician and is

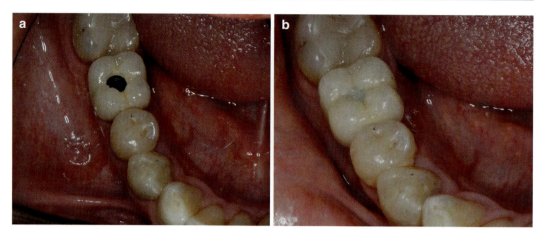

Fig. 7.15 (**a**) Cement-screw-retained restoration is tightened to the implant, and (**b**) access hole is covered with composite

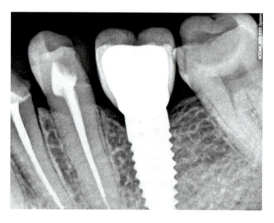

Fig. 7.16 Radiological image shows precise seating of the restoration in the implant

scanned and milled from zirconium (Fig. 7.18a, b). The framework is temporarily cemented to titanium base and checked in the mouth (Figs. 7.19 and 7.20a, b).

Ceramics were veneered on the zirconium frameworks, and they were cemented definitively with adhesive resin cement of titanium bases (Figs. 7.21 and 7.22a, b). Before cementation, the access entrance of the titanium base is covered with wax to protect the basal screw from cement contamination. The occlusal opening must be wide enough that the screw can be rotated without restrictions.

The final step of cement-screw-retained restoration is delivery, where the crowns are screwed onto the implants. Temporary implant-supported crowns are removed, the internal aspect of the implants and soft peri-implant tissues is rinsed with chlorhexidine digluconate solution, and the cement-screw-retained zirconium oxide ceramic restorations are tightened to their respective implants (Fig. 7.23a, b). Radiographic examination was performed to verify the accuracy of the restoration/implant connection (Fig. 7.24).

Occlusal openings are isolated in the following way. First, polytetrafluorethylene tape is packed onto the top of the basal screw until all inner space is filled. Then, hydrofluoric acid is applied to ceramic walls of the screw access tunnel to be etched. Silane, adhesive, and finally composite are applied in succession to close the entrance as esthetically as possible (Fig. 7.25a, b).

Non-hexed Bases for Fixed Partial Dentures

The previous technique can also be applied to fixed partial dentures. The main difference here is that unlike the single crowns where the implant must have an anti-rotation index such as the hexed shape, in the case of fixed bridges, the titanium bases are non-hexed (Figs. 7.26 and 7.27a, b).

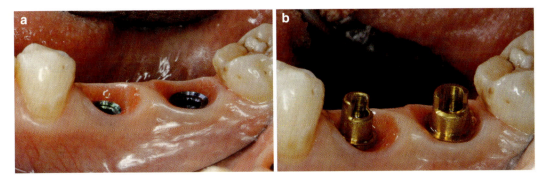

Fig. 7.17 (**a**) The two sites to be restored. (**b**) Titanium bases are tried in the sites prior to developing the wax replica

Fig. 7.18 (**a**) Example of a waxed abutment framework on a titanium base ready to be copy milled. (**b**) Final copy-milled Zirconai abutment framework

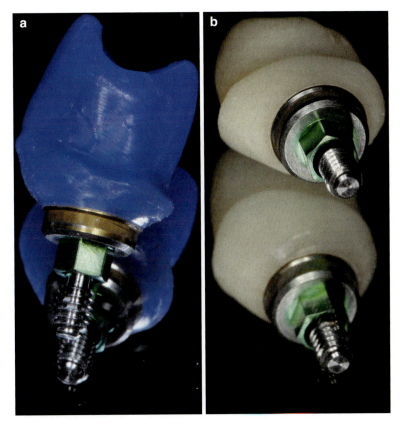

There is a common misconception about the use of non-hexed bases, as it is believed that in the absence of hex indexing, the force transfer mainly rests on the abutment screw; therefore, screw loosening or fracture may be common. The use of screw-retained restorations indeed had more screw loosening, compared to the cemented approach; however, it occurred due to nonpassive frameworks made by casting procedures. Hexed and non-hexed bases have the same conus connection—the contacting plane, where forces are transferred from the abutment to the implant (Fig. 7.28). Hexes are required for the positioning of single restorations and for anti-rotational purposes. When two implants are connected by a fixed partial denture, there is only a single path of insertion for the bridge; therefore, hex is not required. Additionally, the absence of hex indexing allows prosthetic treatment of nonparallel implants. The layer of cement ensures the passivity of such a bridge, as a fixed partial denture is cemented on non-hexed titanium bases and later the entire structure is tightened to the implants.

Cement-screw-retained restoration with non-hexed bases was selected as a restorative option in the case of two integrated implants (Biohorizons, Birmingham, AL, USA). Titanium bases were reduced vertically to fit the interoc-

clusal space; also an indexing groove was made in the lateral side of the base (Fig. 7.29). A zirconium oxide framework was milled, veneered with ceramics, glazed, and cemented on the bases (Fig. 7.30a, b). The restoration is connected to implants; access holes are isolated and closed with composite (Fig. 7.31a–d).

In summary, this is a convenient restorative way to rehabilitate dental implants, particularly if the clinician desires a cement-free solution.

When the demands are such that a cemented option without a screw access opening is to be chosen, the safest, most predictable way of reducing residual excess cement extrusion is to use supragingival abutment margins. Wadhwani et al.

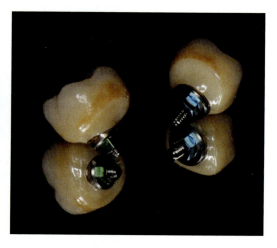

Fig. 7.19 A wax replica modeled by technician is necessary for accurate contour. Then zirconium oxide coping is milled and adapted on the titanium base

Fig. 7.21 The final restorations: these are zirconia crowns cemented onto zirconia frameworks. The zirconia framework has a titanium base

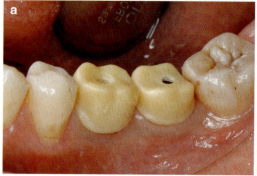
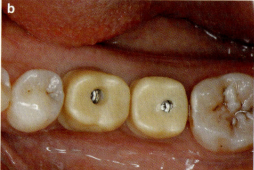

Fig. 7.20 (**a**, **b**) Zirconium coping is temporarily cemented to the titanium base and checked in the mouth

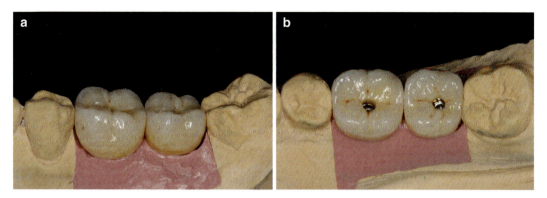

Fig. 7.22 (**a**, **b**) Zirconium oxide ceramic restorations are cemented on titanium bases. Space inside the restoration should be large enough that the basal screw can be rotated passively without restriction

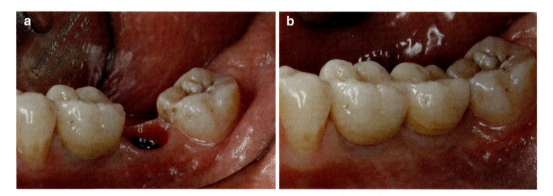

Fig. 7.23 (**a**, **b**) Restorations are tightened to implants with 30 N/cm strength. Radiographic examination shows precise seating of restorations in implants

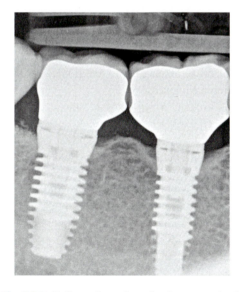

Fig. 7.24 Radiograph confirms fit of crown to implant. Note the peripheral eggshell effect seen as a gap internal to the abutment implant connection (see Chap. 10)

described a technique whereby the addition of pressed ceramics provided an esthetic adhesive abutment margin that could be cemented to the ceramic margin of a restoration.

The Implant Crown with an Esthetic Adhesive Margin (ICEAM)

Techniques have been developed to minimize the extrusion of cement into the peri-implant soft tissues, but it is likely that this problem cannot be predictably eliminated. One major issue when considering excess cement extrusion into the soft tissues around an implant restoration is crown: abutment margin position. The ability to customize an abutment by raising the margins above the soft tissues has been reported. A screw-retained custom metal-ceramic abutment combined with

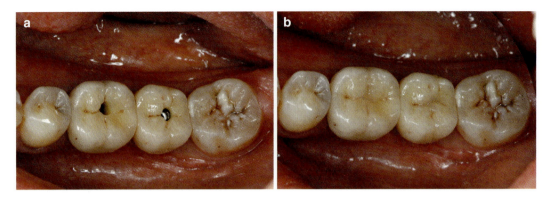

Fig. 7.25 (**a**, **b**) Cement-screw-retained restoration before and after closure of the occlusal openings

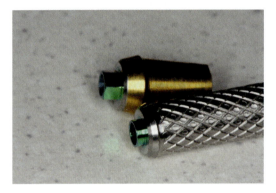

Fig. 7.26 The difference between abutment for single restorations (*yellow* abutment) and base for fixed partial denture. Note the absence of hex indexing, although conus connection is the same in both abutments

an adhesively bonded porcelain restoration was used as a permanent solution to an implant inclination issue combined with a short clinical crown. Traditional porcelain stacking methods produced equigingival and supragingival margins on an abutment to which a porcelain suprastructure was adhesively bonded—a type III veneer. While this technique is innovative, it is time consuming and requires the dental laboratory technician be highly skilled.

Abutment materials can be either metal or ceramic in nature. With the appropriate material selection and conditioning, it is possible to directly wax, then press, porcelain-ceramic mar-

gins to the abutment. Zirconia has been used extensively in dentistry and has gained popularity as an abutment core material due to its strength, white color, and ability to be milled. However, zirconia presents with limitations due to an inherent opacity, poor translucency, and the inability to bond to resin predictably. This is unlike some other ceramic materials that either are susceptible to microabrasion or can be etched, resulting in a more predictable bond with resin materials. A method for overcoming the aforementioned limitations of a zirconia is to add a ceramic margin onto the zirconia abutment. This can be achieved using a fluorapatite glass-ceramic ingot which is pressed onto zirconium oxide. This transitional margin material also improves the esthetics of the abutment yet is less demanding technically compared to traditional ceramic stacking techniques.

The implant crown with an esthetic adhesive margin (ICEAM) is described. It consists of a crown with porcelain butt margin that is bonded to a custom abutment with a pressed porcelain supragingival margin. In a restoration with harmonious margins, the contacting ceramic margins allow for hydrofluoric etching, silane application, and adhesive resin bonding. This type of restoration eliminates some of the disadvantages associated with cement-retained crowns. The ICEAM significantly reduces the amount of excess cement found with traditional

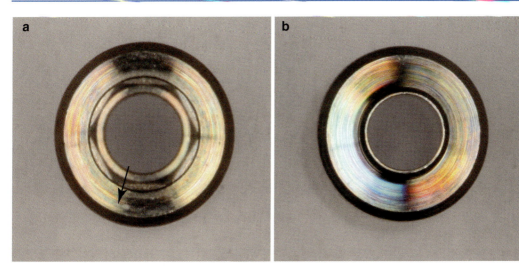

Fig. 7.27 (**a**) Abutment with indexing hex and (**b**) non-hexed abutment. Note that conus connection is the same in both cases. Biohorizon implant

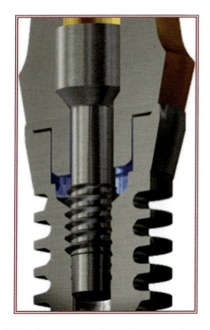

Fig. 7.28 Conus connection: the contacting planes between implant and abutment. There is no actual contact between hex and implant

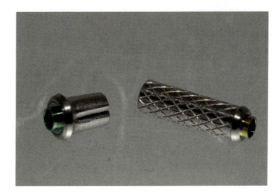

Fig. 7.29 Reduced titanium base with lateral groove

It can help with retention issues found with crown core materials that are problematic with cement adherence, such as zirconia.

Clinical Report

A 60-year-old female patient presented with a transverse fracture through the maxillary right lateral incisor. Clinical and radiographic assessment (Fig. 7.32a, b) indicated the tooth was structurally compromised, and the treatment option selected was extraction and immediate implant placement.

An atraumatic extraction with immediate implant (Bone Level NC, Straumann, Andover,

subgingival margins, allows for direct verification of seating, and enables access to cleaning the cement margins, which is similarly applicable when using metal or ceramic abutment materials.

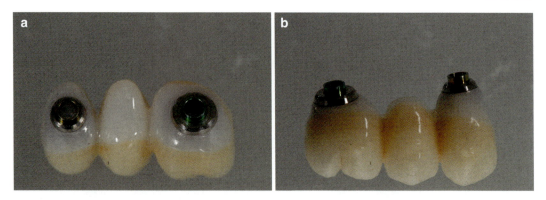

Fig. 7.30 (**a**, **b**) Cement-screw-retained fixed partial denture. Note these are non-indexed (non-hexed titanium bases)

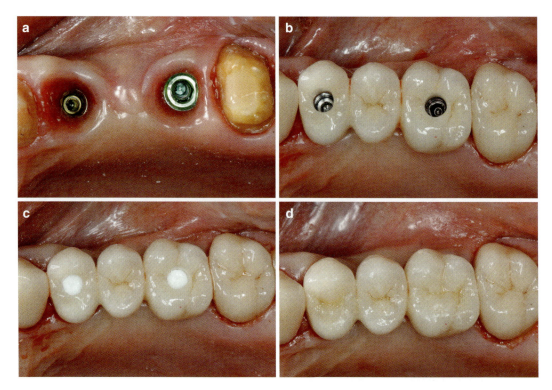

Fig. 7.31 (**a**) Unrestored implants with healing caps removed, ready to receive the fixed cemented-screw-retained fixed partial denture. (**b**) The restoration is placed, confirmed it seats as expected; occlusion adjusted and finally tightened to the prescribed torque value. (**c**) The screws covered first with PTFE tape to protect the integrity of the screwhead, then (**d**) composite, to produce an esthetic result

MA, USA) placement was performed by a periodontist. To minimize the effect of the extraction and implant placement on the soft tissues, the implant was placed slightly toward the palatal aspect. A xenograft material (Bio-Oss, Osteohealth Co., Shirley, NY, USA) was used in the gap between the implant and the bony facial plate. A soft tissue connective tissue graft using an allograft (AlloDerm, LifeCell Co., Branchburg, NJ, USA) was placed out on

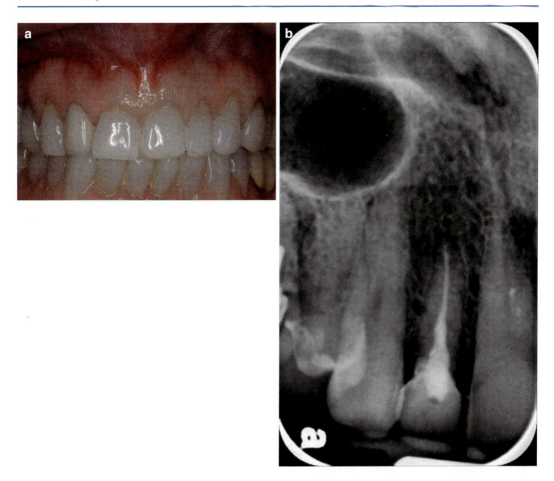

Fig. 7.32 (**a**) Initial photograph and (**b**) radiographs of tooth 7 (right lateral incisor), which has a horizontal fracture

the facial aspect using an envelope technique. To support the gingival tissues during the healing phase, a customized healing abutment was created using a stock temporary abutment (NC Temporary Abutment, Straumann) modified to the contours of the extraction socket site (Fig. 7.33a–c).

Three months after implant placement, the site was deemed ready for restoration. Study casts were obtained along with interocclusal records, facebow recordings (Panadent, Colton, CA, USA), and diagnostic waxing of the tooth. The implant location and soft tissue contour were recorded by fabricating a custom impression coping in a manner first described by

Hinds. This required duplication of the soft tissue contour subgingival to the healing abutment. Duplication of the soft tissue was achieved by removing the customized healing abutment from the implant and attaching it to a laboratory analog (Fig. 7.34a) (NC Analog, Straumann).

An impression of the customized healing abutment/analog complex, similar to that first described by Ken Hinds, was made using a fast-setting vinyl-polysiloxane, or VPS (Blu-Mousse, Parkell, Edgewood, NY, USA), in a copper matrix (Moyco, Moyco Technologies Inc., Montgomeryville, PA, USA), shown in Fig. 7.34b. Once set, the healing abutment was removed from the analog, leaving

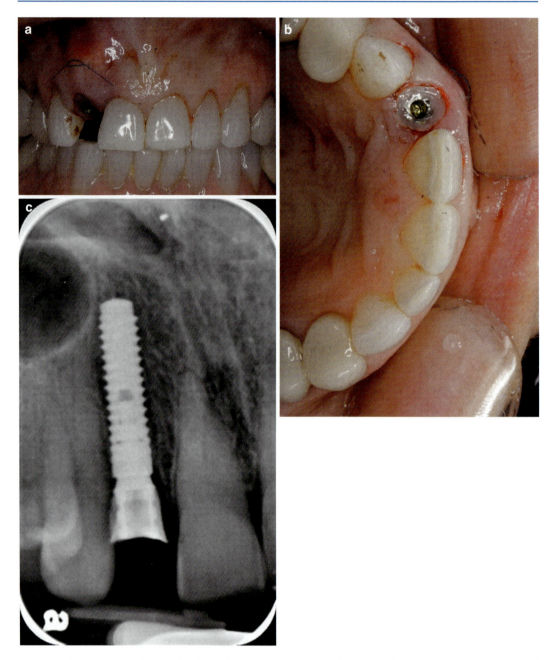

Fig. 7.33 (**a, b**) Photographs and (**c**) radiograph of immediate implant placement following extraction of the fractured tooth

the analog firmly fixed in the VPS material, with the soft tissue contour recorded. An open-tray impression coping was seated onto the laboratory analog, and flowable composite filled the void between it and the VPS imprint made by the customized healing abutment (Fig. 7.35a, b).

To assist in placement throughout the impression procedure, the customized impression coping

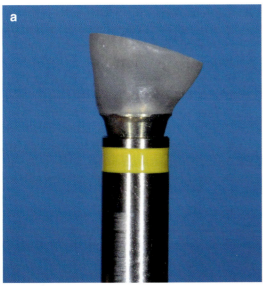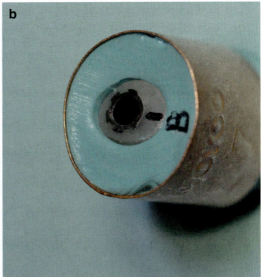

Fig. 7.34 (**a**) Copying the healing abutment contours: custom healing abutment removed from the implant, then attached to a laboratory analog. (**b**) Analog and healing abutment seated into the Blu-Mousse. The orientation is noted. Once set, the healing abutment is unscrewed, leaving the soft tissue contour recorded in the Blu-Mousse

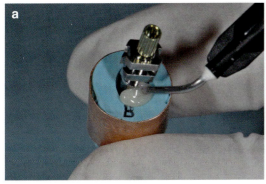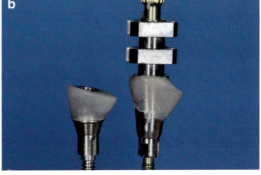

Fig. 7.35 (**a**) Fabrication of custom impression coping. The healing abutment is removed and replaced with a standard impression abutment. Flowable composite is added to the impression abutment, copying the form of the healing abutment. (**b**) Healing abutment and the custom impression coping compared. Both have the same recording of the soft tissue form around the implant

had a buccal location mark placed on it. The custom impression coping was attached to the implant (Fig. 7.36) and a radiograph made to confirm proper seating, and an open-tray implant-level pickup impression was made (Aquasil Ultra, Dentsply, York, PA, USA).

In the laboratory an analog (NC, Straumann, Andover, MA, USA) was attached to the custom impression coping that had been picked up in the impression. A soft tissue gingival mask (Gingitech, Ivoclar Vivadent) was incorporated, and the impression was poured in a type IV stone (Fujirock, GC, Leuven, Belgium).

A wax-up sleeve (Straumann) was modified and fixed to the implant analog and waxed to contour. Then a putty matrix (Sil-Tech, Ivoclar

Vivadent AG, Schaan, Liechtenstein) was made from the diagnostic waxing (Fig. 7.37a). The matrix provided a cutback guide for the abutment framework dimensions needed to support the proposed restoration. The wax pattern incorporating the wax-up sleeve was scanned (Etkon, Straumann), and a CAD/CAM abutment designed and then fabricated in zirconia (Straumann), shown in Fig. 7.37b.

The margins of the zirconia abutment followed the contour of the silicone gingival margin but were placed 1.5 mm subgingival to allow for the proposed pressed margin to have a minimum height of 2 mm. This would allow the pressed porcelain abutment margin to begin at 1.5 mm below the gingival margin and end 0.5 mm supragingivally. The contours of the proposed ceramic

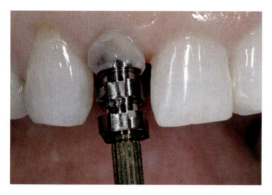

Fig. 7.36 Custom impression coping placed into the implant site. Checked for orientation, before making an open-tray impression

abutment margins were waxed directly to the zirconia abutment and corresponded to the soft tissues that were modeled on the healed soft tissue site (Fig. 7.38a, b).

The waxed zirconia abutment was attached to a sprue and invested in porcelain pressing investment (Microstar HS Investment, Microstar Dental, Lawrenceville, GA, USA). The appropriate shade of ingot was selected (IPS e.max ZirPress, Ivoclar), and the pressing was made following the manufacturer's recommendations in the pressing furnace (Ivopress 5000, Ivoclar Vivadent). The zirconia abutment (Fig. 7.39a, b) with pressed ceramic margin was recovered using airborne particle abrasion with the engaging surfaces of the implant-abutment protected with a layer of wax.

The abutment was used to fabricate a ceramic crown (IPS e.max, Ivoclar Vivadent) of the desired color by fabricating a wax coping crown according to the dimensions dictated by the initial diagnostic waxing, then investing (Microstar HS Investment) and fabricated by the pressing technique described earlier. The porcelain of the crown and zirconia abutment with the pressed porcelain margin was customized with stains and glazed.

The patient approved the esthetic appearance of the restoration, then confirmation of complete seating of the abutment the crown was done with a radiograph prior to cementation. Both the zirconia abutment and IPS e.max crown were returned to the laboratory for conditioning prior to final seat. The fitting surfaces of the abutment's porcelain

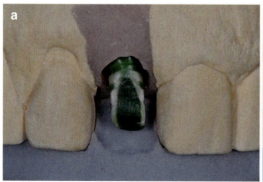
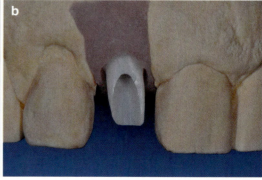

Fig. 7.37 (**a**) For the CAD/CAM process, a scan replica is initially made: wax-up sleeve cut to size and waxed to dimensions according to putty matrix of the original diagnostic waxing. (**b**) CAD/CAM zirconia abutment once fabricated is placed into the original soft tissue cast

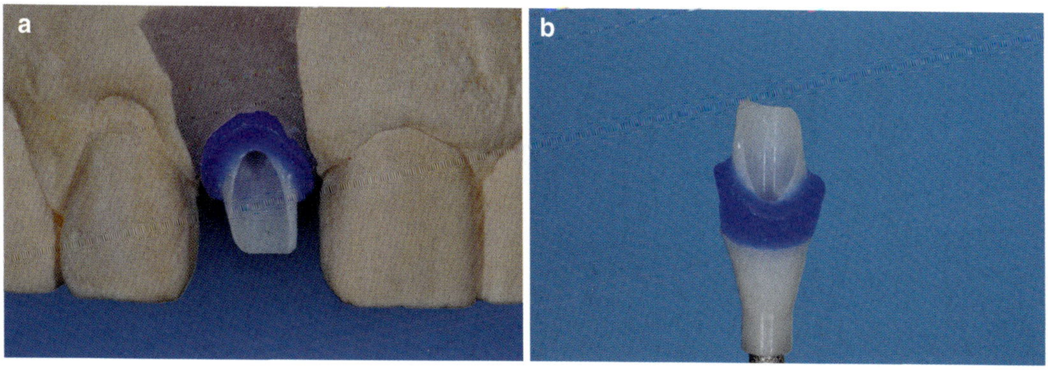

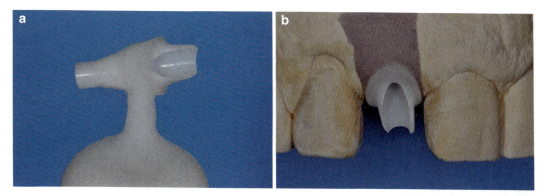

Fig. 7.38 (**a**) Zirconia abutment with wax added to customize and produce a supragingival margin. (**b**) The CAD/CAM zirconia abutment modified with wax

Fig. 7.39 (**a**) Pressing supragingival margin with IPS e.max ZirPress ceramic. The ceramic sprue is still attached. (**b**) Zirconia abutment customized with supragingival pressed porcelain margin

margin and the internal of the ceramic crown were prepared for adhesive bonding by etching with hydrofluoric acid (IPS Ceramic Etching Gel, Ivoclar Vivadent) for 20 s (Fig. 7.40), then rinsed for 20 s. Further cleaning was with 35 % phosphoric acid (Ultra-Etch, Ultradent Products Inc., South Jordan, UT, USA) for 30 s, followed by a 20-s rinse.

Finally, cleaning was completed by separate immersion of the crown and abutment in distilled water in an ultrasonic bath for 5 min. The bonding surfaces were silanated (Silane, Ultradent Products Inc., South Jordan, UT, USA) following thorough oil-free air drying and dried at 100 °C for 5 min in the oven, according to an established protocol for bonding porcelain to porcelain restorations. The zirconia abutment was seated (Fig. 7.41), and the screw was tightened to the appropriate torque (35 Ncm).

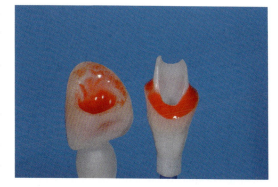

Fig. 7.40 Hydrofluoric conditioning of ceramic bondable surfaces. Both the margins of the abutment and crown, as well as the intaglio of the crown, are susceptible to this process

A small pellet of sterilized polytetrafluoroethylene (PTFE) tape (Oatey Co, Cleveland, OH, USA) was placed into the screw access channel

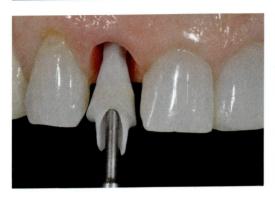

Fig. 7.41 Zirconia abutment with custom-pressed ceramic margin being seated

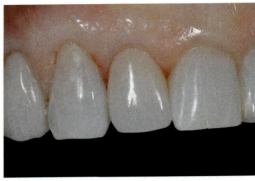

Fig. 7.43 The final implant crown with an esthetic adhesive margin restoration 1 week after cementation

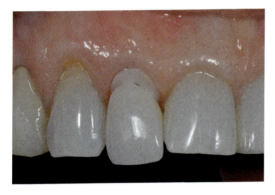

Fig. 7.42 Seating of the IPS e.max crown on the modified zirconia abutment. Note that the margin of the abutment is supragingival

over the screwhead, and the previously etched and silanated supragingival porcelain surfaces were then coated with adhesive resin (Prime and Bond, Dentsply, York, PA, USA) followed by the application of resin luting agent (Ultra Bond Plus, DenMat, Santa Maria, CA, USA). The IPS e.max crown was seated (Fig. 7.42) and held in place for light polymerization.

The final ICEAM was cleaned of excess resin, occlusion evaluated and adjusted, and the crown polished with porcelain polishing points (Dialite, Brasseler USA, Savannah, GA, USA), shown in Fig. 7.43. In many instances the margin can be placed very supragingival especially if the adjacent dentition shows cervical restorations that

will allow for the margin to blend esthetically (Fig. 7.44a, b).

Discussion

Immediate implant placement following atraumatic extraction is considered an acceptable treatment option for the hopeless tooth. Maintaining the soft tissue form after extraction of the tooth remains a challenge due to alveolar housing resorption. One means of accomplishing this is to provide tissue augmentation at the time of implant placement surgery. The implant soft tissue emergence profile can also be established early during the implant healing if an appropriately formed healing abutment is fabricated. This can be copied once osseointegration is confirmed by customizing an impression coping as described in this chapter.

When considering the restorative phase of the treatment, the abutment/crown margin of an implant restoration presents a contentious challenge. By placing this margin subgingival, the transition from the abutment (usually a metal or zirconia substrate) to the crown is hidden, but this exacerbates the issue of excess cement extrusion. This can negatively impact the health and integrity of the implant-supporting tissues. Alternatively, if the junc-

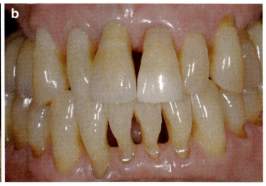

Fig. 7.44 (**a**, **b**) The margin can be placed very supragingival if cervical restorations allow for the margin to blend esthetically

tion is supragingival, the cement issue is negated, but the margin transition becomes visible. One method of overcoming these problems is to use materials for the abutment margin and crown margin that are compatible esthetically and capable of uniting by adhesive bonding. This allows for the margin junction to be placed supragingival. The customization of the abutment and crown components has been previously described; however, the materials and techniques used were that of traditional porcelain stacking followed by sintering the porcelain. This is a very technique-sensitive procedure, as the materials shrink markedly, requiring multiple porcelain application and sintering cycles.

With the introduction of pressed ceramic systems comes the ability to wax directly to the implant-abutment, invest, and then process in porcelain, with minimal dimensional change. The technique is less demanding on the skills of the technician as multiple applications are not required. It can also be more economical as more than one unit can be invested and pressed at the same time. This form of customization with the pressed ceramic systems available today allows for processing directly onto either metal or zirconia substructures. Pressed ceramics also allow the ceramist to be more innovative with other types of implant restoration designs. The pressed

ceramic can also be readily etched with hydrofluoric acid, so the two margin surfaces can be bonded together. This gives an esthetic and almost seamless transition from implant-abutment to cemented coronal restoration, much like that seen with traditional porcelain veneers bonded onto teeth.

Moisture control is an important factor in achieving predicable adhesive bonding. The use of supragingival margins facilitates the ability to control moisture when compared with subgingival margins where sulcular fluid may negatively affect the bonding process.

ICEAM abutments, due to their supragingival design, can also aid in the clinical evaluation of complete seating of the restorations.

Summary for the ICEAM

The ICEAM is a restoration that has several advantages, which include: control of cement lute site that has the potential to reduce cement-induced peri-implant disease, easier cleanup, and the ability to improve adhesion of zirconia abutments. It is an esthetic restoration that can be economically made and is applicable to both metal and ceramic abutment materials capable of being used with pressable ceramic systems. It is considerably less demanding on the laboratory

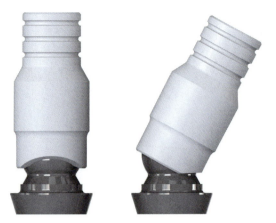

Fig. 7.45 Casting angled abutment (Dynamic Abutment® Solutions, Spain). Designed to allow angle changes within the screw access channel from straight and up to 28°

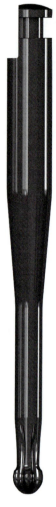

technician compared to other means of creation of a porcelain margin on an abutment.

New Innovations from the Implant Manufacturers

Some implant manufacturers are now designing and developing angled abutments, such as those shown in Fig. 7.45 (dynamic abutments), allowing for screw-retained options to be used in sites where this would be problematic with a straight abutment form. The screwdriver allows for angle changes in some instances up to 30°, by having a round engaging end (Fig. 7.46). The abutments have an internal curved flute that allows the screw to change angulation as it is placed, and the driver can then engage the screwhead at multiple angles, allowing the correct torque value to be applied (Fig. 7.47). Design concepts such as the angled screw channel abutment will allow the technician

Fig. 7.46 The screwdriver has a "ball"-type end, allowing it to engage the screwhead from many angles

more flexibility in where the screw access channel will emerge, thus reducing the problem of esthetics and occlusal loading sites.

Fig. 7.47 Angled screw channel abutment (Nobel Biocare, Switzerland) is a zirconia CAD/CAM abutment; it allows angle deviations up to and including 25°

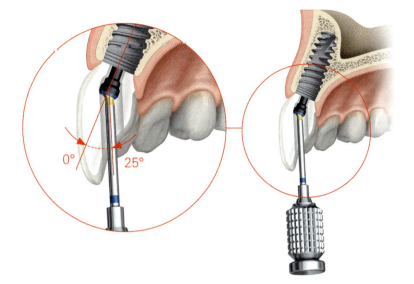

Conclusion

Several techniques have been developed from the implant restorative design perspective to eliminate cement extrusion into the tissues. Placing a cemented, bonded margin that is supragingival would likely minimize cement extrusion into the tissues. Completely eliminating cement is also a possibility by utilizing screw retention. This can be done with high esthetic value and complete control of the occlusion. Where the implant angulation is such that the straight-line access would be undesirable, newer screw access channel angled abutments can also be considered.

Bibliography

Agar JR, Cameron SM, Hughbanks JC, Parker MH. Cement removal from restorations luted to titanium abutments with simulated subgingival margins. J Prosthet Dent. 1997;78:43–7.

Chen ST, Darby IB, Reynolds EC. A prospective clinical study of non-submerged immediate implants: clinical outcomes and esthetic results. Clin Oral Implants Res. 2007;18:552–62.

Christensen GJ. Margin fit of gold inlay castings. J Prosthet Dent. 1966;16:297–305.

Dumbrigue HB, Abanomi AA, Cheng LL. Techniques to minimize excess luting agent in cement-retained implant restorations. J Prosthet Dent. 2002;87:112–4.

Gapski R, Neugeboren N, Pomeranz AZ, Reissner MW. Endosseous implant failure influenced by crown cementation: a clinical case report. Int J Oral Maxillofac Implants. 2008;23:943–6.

Hebel KS, Gajjar RC. Cement-retained versus screw-retained implant restorations: achieving optimal occlusion and esthetics in implant dentistry. J Prosthet Dent. 1997;77:28–35.

Hinds KF. Custom impression coping for an exact registration of the healed tissue in the esthetic implant restoration. Int J Periodontics Restorative Dent. 1997;17(6):584–91.

Jemt T. Cemented CeraOne and porcelain fused to TiAdapt abutment single-implant crown restorations: a 10 year comparative follow-up study. Clin Implant Dent Relat Res. 2009;11:303–10.

Kan JY, Rungcharassaeng K, Morimoto T, Lozada J. Facial gingival tissue stability after connective tissue graft with single immediate tooth replacement in the esthetic zone: consecutive case report. J Oral Maxillofac Surg. 2009;67(11 Suppl):40–8.

Kano SC, Binon P, Bonfante G, Curtis DA. Effect of casting procedures on screw loosening in UCLA-type abutments. J Prosthodont. 2006;15:1–5.

Linkevicius T, Vindasiute E, Puisys A, Peciuliene V. The influence of margin location on the amount of undetected cement excess after delivery of cement-retained implant restorations. Clin Oral Implants Res. 2011; 22:1379–84.

Magne P, Magne M, Jovanovic SA. An esthetic solution for single-implant restorations—type III porcelain veneer bonded to a screw-retained custom abutment: a clinical report. J Prosthet Dent. 2008;99:2–7.

Michalakis KX, Hirayama H, Garefis PD. Cement-retained versus screw-retained implant restorations: a critical review. Int J Oral Maxillofac Implants. 2003;18: 719–28.

Moráguez OD, Belser UC. The use of polytetrafluoroethylene tape for the management of screw access channels in implant-supported prostheses. J Prosthet Dent. 2010;103:189–91.

Nissan J, Narobai D, Gross O, Ghelfan O, Chaushu G. Long-term outcome of cemented versus screw-retained implant-supported partial restorations. Int J Oral Maxillofac Implants. 2011;26:1102–7.

Pauletto N, Lahiffe BJ, Walton JN. Complications associated with excess cement around crowns on osseointegrated implants: a clinical report. Int J Oral Maxillofac Implants. 1999;14(6):865–8.

Rajan M, Gunaseelan R. Fabrication of a cement- and screw-retained implant prosthesis. J Prosthet Dent. 2004;92:578–80.

Schwedhelm ER, Lepe X, Aw TC. A crown venting technique for the cementation of implant-supported crowns. J Prosthet Dent. 2003;89:89–90.

Taylor TD, Agar JR. Twenty years of progress in implant prosthodontics. J Prosthet Dent. 2002;88:89–95.

Theoharidou A, Petridis HP, Tzannas K, Garefis P. Abutment screw loosening in single-implant restorations: a systematic review. Int J Oral Maxillofac Implants. 2008;23:681–90.

Wadhwani C, Piñeyro A. Technique for controlling the cement for an implant crown. J Prosthet Dent. 2009;102:57–8.

Wadhwani C, Hess T, Faber T, Piñeyro A, Chen CS. A descriptive study of the radiographic density of implant restorative cements. J Prosthet Dent. 2010;103:295–302.

Wadhwani C, Piñeyro A, Avots J. An esthetic solution to the screw-retained implant restoration: introduction to the implant crown adhesive plug: clinical report. J Esthet Restor Dent. 2011;23:138–43.

Wadhwani CP, Piñeyro A, Akimoto K. An introduction to the implant crown with an esthetic adhesive margin (ICEAM). J Esthet Restor Dent. 2012;24(4):246–54.

Weber HP, Kim DM, Ng MW, Hwang JW, Fiorellini JP. Peri-implant soft-tissue health surrounding cement- and screw-retained implant restorations: a multi-center, 3-year prospective study. Clin Oral Implants Res. 2006;17:375–9.

Wilson TG. The positive relationship between excess cement and peri-implant disease: a prospective clinical endoscopic study. J Periodontol. 2009;80:1388–92.

Clinical Solutions: PTFE

8

Chandur P.K. Wadhwani

Abstract

Controlling the amount of cement used for the restoration and abutment form is a simple and effective means of reducing residual excess cement. Polytetrafluoroethylene (PTFE), also known as "plumber's tape," has a thickness of close to 50 μm, and it has numerous applications in dentistry. Used as a throwaway spacer, it can limit the amount of cement applied internally within a crown, allowing the cement to be evenly spread on all walls with almost the ideal amount. Used within the abutment itself as a screw head protector, PTFE has proven antimicrobial properties. Techniques such as the PTFE "bib" protector are also described in detail.

Introduction

This chapter deals with some clinical solutions on how to control cement for specific abutment forms. Essentially, the custom copy abutment, a "throwaway" plunger device, will evenly spread a layer of cement almost the exact thickness required on the internal aspect of the restoration. Like all techniques, this has limitations that must be understood. It can really only be used for closed-off abutment systems as it would not provide sufficient cement for an open abutment where cement is expected to flow internally.

The chapter also reports on the use of polytetrafluoroethylene (PTFE) also known as Teflon tape and plumber's tape. As a material, PTFE has one of the lowest coefficients of friction. It is widely used in medicine as a graft material and in dentistry as a suture material, as well as a flossing material. It has applications in restoring implants as well as teeth, which will also be described in this chapter.

Clinical Techniques to Control the Flow and Amount of Cement: The Custom Copy Abutment

The custom copy abutment can be utilized to control and minimize the flow of cement. Loading the abutment with appropriate amount of cement for the system is a simple way to accomplish this. The following text describes how and why this is so useful.

C.P.K. Wadhwani, BDS, MSD
Department of Restorative Dentistry, University of Washington School of Dentistry, Seattle, WA, USA

Private Practice Limited to Prosthodontics, 1200, 116th Ave NE #A, Bellevue, WA 98004, USA
e-mail: cpkw@uw.edu

C.P.K. Wadhwani (ed.), *Cementation in Dental Implantology: An Evidence-Based Guide*, DOI 10.1007/978-3-642-55163-5_8, © Springer-Verlag Berlin Heidelberg 2015

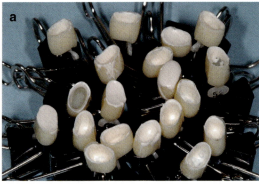

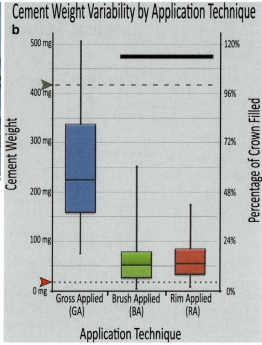

Fig. 8.1 (**a**) Actual photo of how some dentists loaded crowns with cement as if they were to be placed on implants in their offices. (**b**) Mean and range of cement used with different application techniques (Used with permission from Wadhwani et al. (2012). Copyright © Quintessence Publishing Company, Inc., Chicago, IL, USA)

Cementation Techniques

Clinicians often do not understand that only a very limited amount of cement is needed to fix a restoration to an implant abutment. A recent survey of more than 400 dentists showed that many dentists placed in excess of 20 times more cement into the crown than was required (Fig. 8.1a, b). This overload of cement means that 95 % is extruded out at the restorative margin, which is frequently situated below the gum, making cement removal virtually impossible.

Solution

Understanding how much cement is needed for an individual restoration is paramount if residual excess cement extrusion is to be avoided. An "ideal" volume of cement can be calculated if the size of the abutment is known and how it compares to the internal dimensions of the crown that is to be seated onto it.

When fabricating tooth-borne restorations such as full coverage crowns, the technician will frequently apply a die spacer material. This provides relief space for the cement lute. The crown is therefore fabricated on a die that is larger than the actual prepared tooth. The space provided for cement on the inside of the crown during the making of the crown is the same thickness as a layer of nail polish approximately 50 μm thick, which is about the thickness of a human hair!

When an implant restoration is made to be cemented over an abutment, the crown or bridge has a relief space provided in a similar manner. In the case of the CAD/CAM restoration, this is usually milled into the restoration. Some implant companies make laboratory analogs, which are inclusive of the abutment (Straumann solid abutment). These abutments are larger in size than the actual implant abutment used in the patient. The larger dimension of the laboratory analog is advantageous to the technician, as he or she does not have to apply additional spacer material.

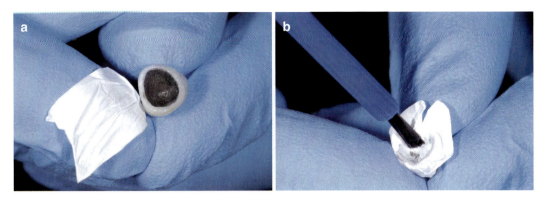

Fig. 8.2 (**a**) A piece of PTFE ready to be adapted to the inside of the crown. This has Vaseline painted internally. (**b**) A dry paintbrush is used to fully adapt the PTFE

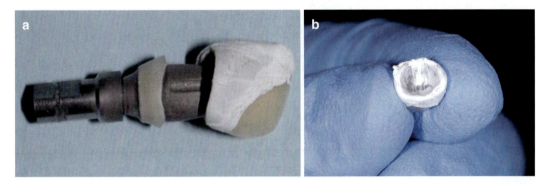

Fig. 8.3 (**a**) The abutment is gently seated if the PTFE requires further adaptation. (**b**) The inside of the crown has a layer of PTFE tape adapted to it

A technique has been developed using a spacer and some fast-setting dental impression material to make a Chairside Copy Abutment (CCA) that can be used to coat the inside of the crown with a layer of cement approximating to the 50 μm needed.

The first stage: The crown is painted internally with Vaseline or a water-soluble lubricant. This allows polytetrafluoroethylene (PTFE) (plumber's tape, which is 50 μm thick) to be adapted to, and stick to, the inside of the crown using a dry brush (Fig. 8.2a, b). The adaptation is completed by gently pushing the abutment into the crown and then carefully removing it (Fig. 8.3a).

To make the CCA use a fast-setting impression or bite registration material. Fill the inside of the crown and continue to overfill until a "handle" is produced (Fig. 8.4a, b). Hint: use a fine-tip nozzle. Then allow the material to set (Fig. 8.5).

Remove the CCA, and then remove the PTFE and discard. Thoroughly clean the inside of the crown (important!) to remove the lubricating agent (Fig. 8.6). Now you have a chairside copy abutment. The CCA is 50 μm smaller than the inside of the crown. Inspect it, compare it to the actual abutment, and make sure you know the orientation (Fig. 8.7).

The CCA is now ready for use. Place the abutment in the patient's mouth, confirm that it seats correctly, and then torque the screw to the appropriate preload value. The crown is now ready to be cemented. Load the crown with more cement than is required. When CCA is pushed into the crown and seated fully, the excess cement will be extruded chairside and easily

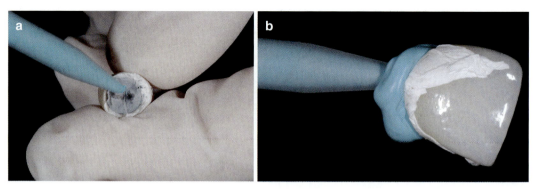

Fig. 8.4 (**a**) Making the CCA. The crown with the PTFE lining is being filled with Blu-Mousse. (**b**) A handle is being formed

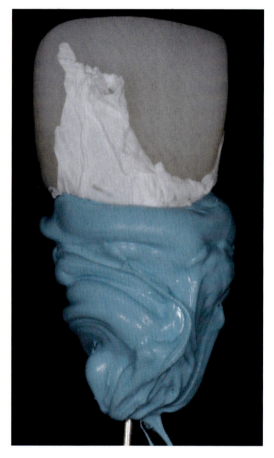

Fig. 8.5 The completed Blu-Mousse replica is allowed to set

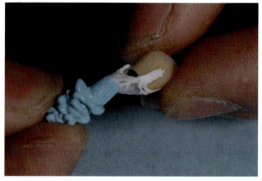

Fig. 8.6 Remove the Blu-Mousse copy abutment, take out the PTFE and discard, and then follow with thorough cleaning of the crown

plunger, extruding excess cement. It is now discarded and the inside of the crown should have an even amount of cement lining it. If there is a deficiency, add a minimal amount. The crown is seated intraorally (Fig. 8.10) with almost no excess cement, maintaining health and reducing cleanup time. Cleanup should be absolutely minimal.

On completion, it is advised to make a post-cementation radiograph to confirm both that the crown has been seated correctly and that no excess cement exists—that is, provided the cement used is radio-opaque enough!

removed—this is done outside of the mouth (Figs. 8.8a, b and 8.9).

The Blu-Mousse (Bite registration material, Parkell, Edgewood, NY, USA) CCA has acted as a

Advantages of the CCA

A fast, inexpensive, simple technique, this approach limits excess cement to an absolute

Fig. 8.7 Comparing the real abutment to the CCA, confirm orientation and check for defects

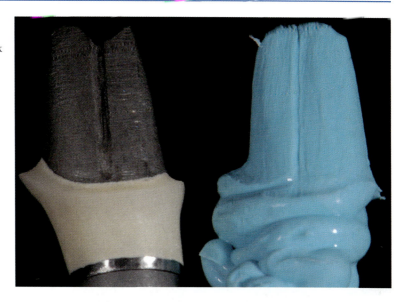

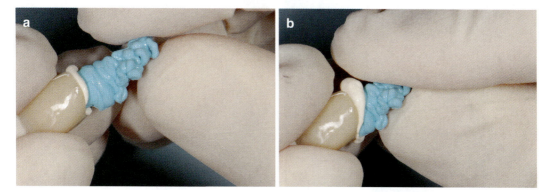

Fig. 8.8 (**a**) The CCA is gently seated at first, (**b**) then completely pushed into the crown, allowing excess to be removed extraorally. Hint: when you first try this, use cement with an extended setting time

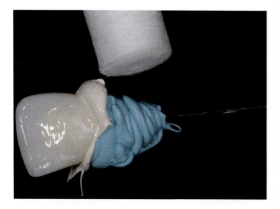

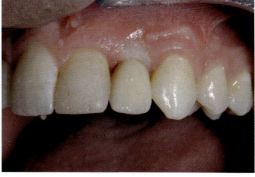

Fig. 8.10 The crown is seated onto the abutment. Cleanup is minimal (Note blanching is from the abutment, which has a 360° porcelain supragingival margin)

Fig. 8.9 Once fully seated, the excess cement is removed

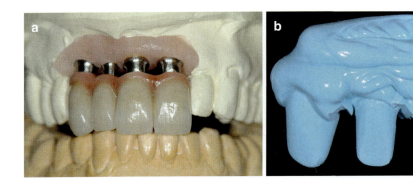

Fig. 8.11 (**a**) This four-unit cemented prosthesis had a (**b**) copy custom abutment device made to pre-extrude excess cement. It was fabricated in a similar manner as the CCA using PTFE as a spacer providing 50 μm lute space

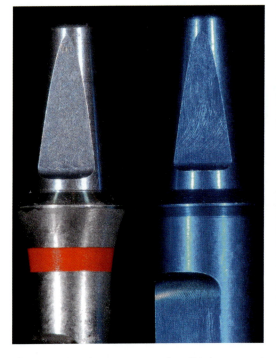

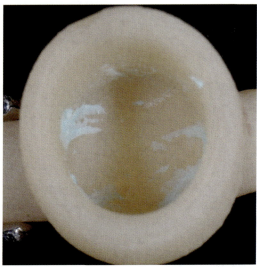

Fig. 8.13 A vinylpolysiloxane (VPS) material has been placed directly into this crown. On removal, residue is noted. This could interfere with the cementing process and must be considered undesirable

Fig. 8.12 These images represent the solid abutment and its laboratory analog (*blue*). Although they appear the same size, the analog is larger in dimension by approximately 20 μm. If it is used as a pre-extrusion device, insufficient cement will line the walls of the restoration

minimum and makes cleanup quicker and easier. The CCA can be used for custom, stock, and even multiple abutments (Fig. 8.11a, b).

Variations to this type of copy abutment have been described but, in the author's opinion, may present more problems, as the ideal amount of space for cement has not been factored into their design. One such example is to use the laboratory abutment the restoration was fabricated on. Most have a built-in die spacer and so are physically larger than the true abutment, so when they are used to pre-extrude cement and distribute the cement onto the crown walls, they frequently underload the crown. Too much cement is extruded (Fig. 8.12).

Direct fabrication of a copy abutment without the PTFE spacer being used has several potential issues. First, the material being used to fabricate the vinylpolysiloxane (VPS) abutment may leave a residue within the crown (Fig. 8.13).

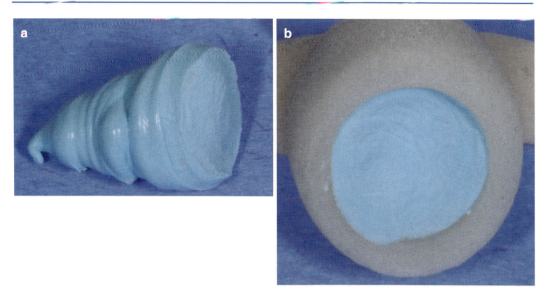

Fig. 8.14 (**a**) This VPS abutment was fabricated without the PTFE spacer. It fractured on attempted removal; (**b**) the other part had to be removed from the inside of the crown

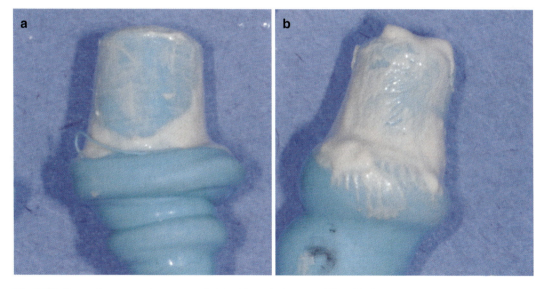

Fig. 8.15 Comparing a copy abutment made (**a**) without the PTFE and (**b**) with the spacer. Note the distribution of the cement on the abutment—this is mirrored by the internal spread of cement lute within the restoration

Secondly, with no spacer, if any undercuts or irregularities exist inside the crown, they may lock the VPS material in place, and the copy abutment will be difficult to remove without fracturing (Fig. 8.14a, b).

Finally, if a VPS copy abutment is made without a spacer, the fit of the copy abutment would be very close. This has a tendency to push the cement up into the occlusal aspect of the crown, an undesirable position for cement flow, leaving the walls of the crown almost bare of cement (Fig. 8.15a, b). Understanding how cement placed primarily in the occlusal aspect (Chap. 4) produces cement extrusion with greater force than when evenly distributed also gives cause for concern.

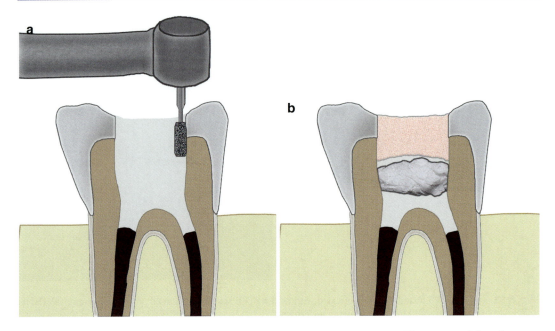

Fig. 8.16 (**a**) Diagram of the experiment design. Endodontic access prepared and teeth sterilized. (**b**) The teeth were disinfected, rubber dam placed, and an end-odontic access cavity cut. The test materials to be compared: cotton wool or PTFE were placed within the pulp chamber and 4 mm of Cavit placed to seal the cavity

Other Uses of PTFE Tape in Dentistry

PTFE has been used as a spacer within the screw access channel to protect the implant abutment screw. Traditionally cotton wool was used; however, when this material becomes contaminated, it gives off a disagreeable odor. PTFE does not. The author is currently evaluating the antibacterial properties of this material when it remains within the abutment.

An in vitro study was conducted by the Endodontic and Microbiology Department of the University of Washington and the author and published in *Quintessence International*. This was an evaluation of the ability to resist bacterial colonization of sterilized PTFE pellets versus sterilized cotton wool pellets that are used as a spacer in endodontics.

Twenty-six molar teeth had endodontic access cavities cut and the contents of the pulp removed. They were disinfected externally and internally using sodium hypochlorite then sterilized using an autoclave (Fig. 8.16a, b). Six teeth were used as controlled pairs: three used cotton wool pellets, and three used PTFE pellets. They were sealed with the zinc oxide/eugenol (Cavit) and immersed in sterile

media. They were used to confirm no bacterial contamination was derived from the tooth itself. The test teeth, 10 in each group, were similarly treated, but after sealing, they were immersed in a media broth seeded with *Streptococcus gordonii* and incubated for 7 days (Fig. 8.17).

Once removed, the molar teeth were washed with disinfectant, and the area around the temporary restoration was thoroughly cleaned so as not to contaminate the test sites. The Cavit material was removed carefully and the test spacers, cotton wool, and PTFE retrieved. These were then sealed in individual Eppendorf tubes with 1 ml of media broth and agitated to dislodge adherent bacteria. The broth and spacers were then placed on agar plates and incubated under anaerobic conditions for 48 h. *S. gordonii* contamination of the spacer material was evaluated by the presence of colonies on the agar plates (Fig. 8.18).

The results showed that nine out of ten teeth had bacterial growth associated with them when cotton wool was used as a spacer. This compared to only one out of ten in the PTFE group (Fig. 8.19). When the only tooth with growth from the PTFE group was rechecked, it was found to be contaminated and possibly had a crack that extended from outside the tooth to the pulp cham-

Fig. 8.17 Schematic representation of the experimental setup (Reprinted with permission from Quintessence International 2012)

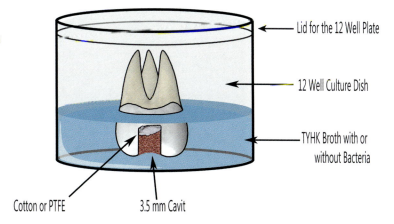

Lid for the 12 Well Plate

12 Well Culture Dish

TYHK Broth with or without Bacteria

Cotton or PTFE   3.5 mm Cavit

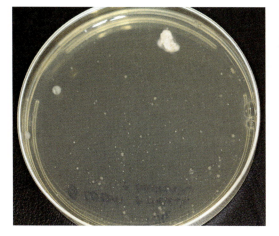

Fig. 8.18 Example of agar plate with cotton wool pellet, demonstrating *S. gordonii* contamination; 9/10 showed similar contamination

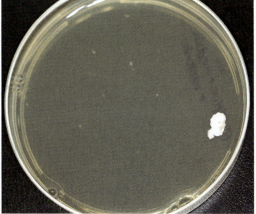

Fig. 8.19 Example of PTFE spacer. This showed no colony growth (specks are air voids within agar media) in 9/10 cultures, demonstrating inhibition of bacterial growth

ber. This study demonstrated that PTFE was a superior spacer compared to cotton wool in teeth and was attributed to the following: PTFE is not an organic material like cotton, so its use as a bacterial substrate is limited. The low coefficient of friction may inhibit adherence of bacteria and so prevent establishment of bacterial colonies.

Although the use of the PTFE inside implants is still under investigation, it has been used by the author for many years now and has performed very well. The material is acquired from a hardware store and cut into 15 cm strips, then placed within an autoclavable bag. This allows for sterilization (Fig. 8.20).

Pellets are formed by cutting a strip of the tape 1 cm in length and rolling between gloved fingers. The pellet can then be introduced into the screw access chamber to protect the screw head from cement blockage that may prevent the driver engaging it in the future if required (Fig. 8.21a, b). It is easily found and recovered when necessary.

It has also been used as a "bib" to reduce cement contamination from oral crevicular fluids and to assist in protecting the oral mucosa from potential irritation from chemicals found in cement

This technique uses a 2–3 mm length of sterilized PTFE. A rubber dam punch provides a hole in the center of the tape. The implant abutment is carefully placed into the PTFE, which is slipped up but not beyond the cement margin. This must be carefully executed so as not to get the tape trapped when the abutment is screwed into the implant and also not to trap the PTFE tape within the cemented margin itself (Figs. 8.22a, b and 8.23a, b).

Fig. 8.20 PTFE comes in the form of a spool. It is cut into convenient-size strips, placed in an autoclave bag, and sterilized

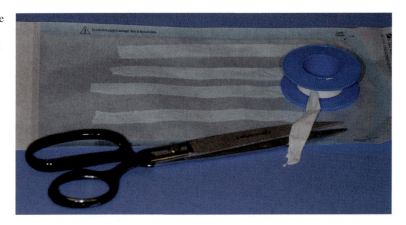

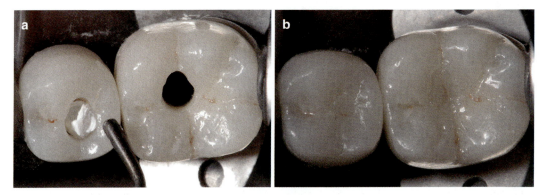

Fig. 8.21 (**a**) Sterilized PTFE pellet being placed into the screw access chamber of a screw-retained implant crown (ICAP). (**b**) The tape protects the screw head under the inlay plug

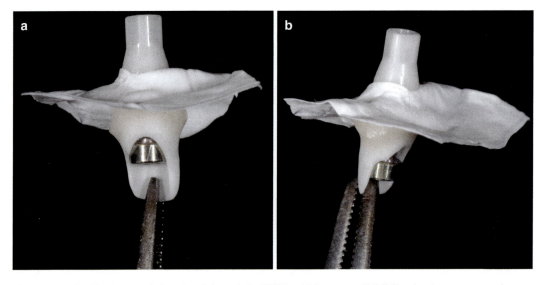

Fig. 8.22 (**a**, **b**) The abutment being placed through the PTFE, which acts as a "bib." Care is taken not to trap the tape at either the implant engaging or the cemented margin site

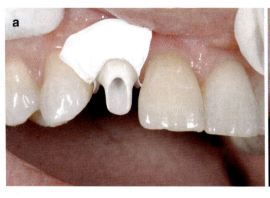
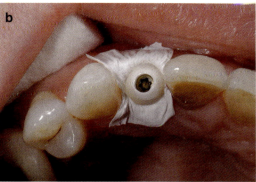

Fig. 8.23 (**a**) Facial and (**b**) occlusal view of the PTFE bib

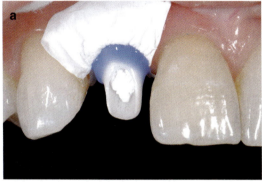
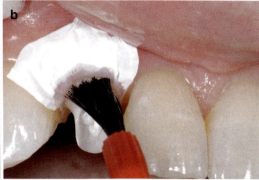

Fig. 8.24 (**a**) The PTFE used to prevent phosphoric acid gel irritating the tissue. This is used to clean the porcelain and decontaminate from effects of saliva just prior to cementation. (**b**) Application of a silane conditioner. Note the PTFE pellet used to prtect the screw head

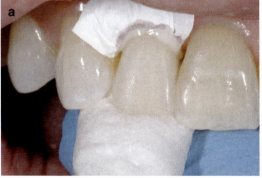
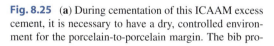
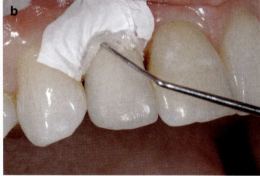

Fig. 8.25 (**a**) During cementation of this ICAAM excess cement, it is necessary to have a dry, controlled environment for the porcelain-to-porcelain margin. The bib protects the site. (**b**) On cement set, the bib is easily removed along with excess cement

Although a rubber dam is preferred, it is not always possible to place one. The bib provides an adequate barrier, seen here being used on a lateral incisor site implant. Note the margins of this abutment are supragingival, and the PTFE tape lies apical to the margin (Fig. 8.24a, b).

The bib both protects the soft tissues and isolates the restorative field. It is inexpensive and easy to use, but care must be exercised so as not to trap it either at the abutment screw site or at the cemented margin (Figs. 8.25a, b and 8.26).

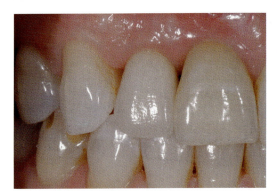

Fig. 8.26 Immediately after cementation, the tissues have not been damaged by chemical insult, and the site has been controlled with respect to contamination

Conclusion

Simple, yet effective, clinical techniques have been developed that utilize a material designed for industry—PTFE tape. This material has properties that can aid implant restoration. As a spacer to prevent cement from locking out the screw head within the abutment, it has proven antimicrobial properties and is also inexpensive and easily removed. As a liner prior to making a disposable custom copy abutment, the use of PTFE tape provides a cement space that is ideal—50 μm. When used as a bib around a cemented abutment margin, it can help isolate a site, minimizing contamination.

Bibliography

Chee WW, Duncan J, Afshar M, Moshaverinia A. Evaluation of the amount of excess cement around the margins of cement-retained dental implant restorations: the effect of the cement application method. J Prosthet Dent. 2013;109(4):216–21.

Dumbrigue HB, Abanomi AA, Cheng LL. Techniques to minimize excess luting agent in cement-retained implant restorations. J Prosthet Dent. 2002;87(1): 112–4.

Hess TA. A technique to eliminate subgingival cement adhesion to implant abutments by using polytetrafluoroethylene tape. J Prosthet Dent. 2014;112(2):365–8.

Moráguez OD, Belser UC. The use of polytetrafluoroethylene tape for the management of screw access channels in implant-supported prostheses. J Prosthet Dent. 2010;103(3):189–91.

Paranjpe A, Jain S, Alibhai KJ, Wadhwani CP, Darveau RP, Johnson JD. In vitro microbiologic evaluation of PTFE and cotton as spacer materials. Quintessence Int. 2012;43(8):703–7.

Wadhwani C, Piñeyro A. Technique for controlling the cement for an implant crown. J Prosthet Dent. 2009; 102(1):57–8.

Wadhwani CP, Piñeyro AF. Implant cementation: clinical problems and solutions. Dent Today. 2012;31(1):56. 58, 60–2.

Wadhwani C, Hess T, Piñeyro A, Opler R, Chung KH. Cement application techniques in luting implant-supported crowns: a quantitative and qualitative survey. Int J Oral Maxillofac Implants. 2012;27(4): 859–64.

Importance of the Implant Screw Access Channel Location: Development of a Screw Access Channel Locating Device and Radiographic Integrator

9

Chandur P.K. Wadhwani, Tony Daher, Kevin C. Lin, and Richard M. Opler

Abstract

There are occasions when the implant restoration requires removal. Cemented restorations may not allow easy removal. The clinician may then be presented with the challenge of accessing the abutment screw channel with a bur. This chapter deals with several ways to provide information that could be useful in determining where the access cavity should be made. These may expedite the procedure and limit any damage as a result, saving time and, potentially, expense.

C.P.K. Wadhwani, BDS (Hons), MSD (✉)
Department of Restorative Dentistry, University of Washington School of Dentistry, Seattle, WA, USA

Private Practice Limited to Prosthodontics, 1200, 116th Ave NE #A, Bellevue, WA 98004, USA
e-mail: cpkw@uw.edu

T. Daher, DDS, MSEd
Department of Restorative Dentistry, Loma Linda University, School of Dentistry, LaVerne, CA, USA

Department of Restorative Dentistry, Loma Lina University, Private Practice Limited to Prosthodontics, LaVerne, CA, USA

K.C. Lin, DDS
Department of Integrated Reconstructive Dental Sciences, University of the Pacific, Arthur A. Dugoni School of Dentistry, San Francisco, CA, USA

R.M. Opler, BA, DDS
Department of Senior Dental Student, University of Washington School of Dentistry, Seattle, WA, USA

Introduction

Cemented implant restorations have many advantages associated with their use. However, should the restoration require removal, this may be problematic and unpredictable.

Abutment screw loosening under a cement-retained implant restoration presents one of the most challenging issues to the implant dentist. From the initial concept of cemented restorations in 1990, retrievability has been discussed with special focus concerning the ability to access the abutment screw. Instances in which access to the underlying screw channel are useful include screw loosening, repair of the restoration, and improving access to the implant body for hygiene or treatment of peri-implant disease (Fig. 9.1).

If the crown can be predictably, temporarily cemented in a manner that allows for retrieval, there is no issue. However, most US dental schools

C.P.K. Wadhwani (ed.), *Cementation in Dental Implantology: An Evidence-Based Guide*, DOI 10.1007/978-3-642-55163-5_9, © Springer-Verlag Berlin Heidelberg 2015

surveyed in 2010 were found to cement the implant restoration definitively, with the result that when the crown needs to be removed, this may be difficult, if not impossible, to accomplish. The only solution left is to evaluate the screw access site, cut into the crown, and locate the abutment screw.

Current Methods of Recording the Implant Screw Access Site

The need to evaluate the location of the underlying screw access site has led to the development of several techniques. However, all of these

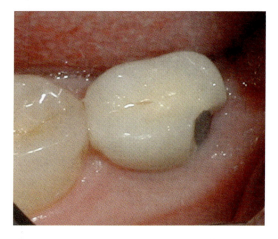

Fig. 9.1 Fractured porcelain on this restoration necessitates removal and possible repair

(described below) have deficiencies associated with them. They all require some level of guesswork, which may result in excessive destruction of the restoration, damage to the abutment, and, in some instances, destruction to the implant itself (Fig. 9.2). Most are also considered time consuming, due to the lack of three-dimensional information given.

The point of entry for the drill must be assessed by one of the following:

1. Arbitrarily, that is, guesstimate. The crown provides little, if any, clue as to where the screw channel lies or even the extent and the form of the supporting abutment (Fig. 9.3).
2. Evaluating a radiograph of the site—a technique frequently employed when accessing a pulp chamber in a natural tooth during endodontic therapy. This may provide approximate information as to mesial-distal location of the implant and may provide clues to the shape of the abutment if the crown is not extensively radiopaque (Figs. 9.4 and 9.5).
3. Pre-cementation photographic documentation—giving a two-dimensional picture of a 3D site (Fig. 9.6a–c).
4. Have the dental laboratory tattoo on the crown. However, the patient may object, especially in the anterior (Fig. 9.7).
5. Make putty indexes—find the hole approximate, add wax, then index.

Fig. 9.2 The restoration has been removed. The underlying abutment is damaged by overpreparation of the screw access hole. The abutment required replacement, needlessly increasing the cost of the replacement restoration

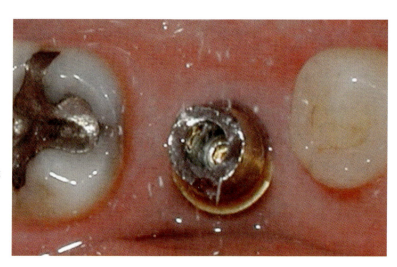

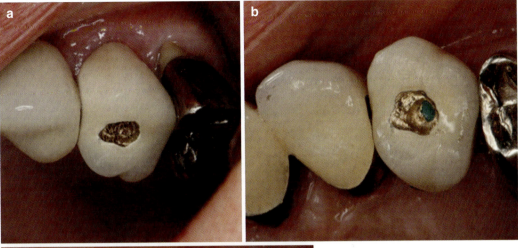

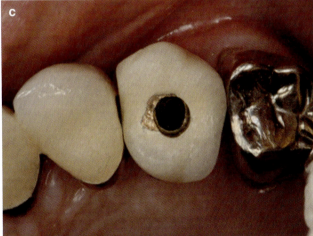

Fig. 9.3 (**a**) Initial access to the screw channel is determined by "best guess" of the site and angulation. (**b**) Often a large area is involved. (**c**) More extensive destruction of the crown frequently occurs

6. Have the dental laboratory make individual vacuum guides. It requires special materials (vacuum former) and requires a complete cast to fabricate upon. If the adjacent dentition requires any restorative work or if teeth move, then it cannot be modified easily (Fig. 9.8).

7. Use computer-aided design (CAD) and computer-aided machined (CAM) technology (look at an existing digital image used to design and fabricate the abutment, then guesstimate). Limited to CAD/CAM abutments and crowns that have stored images available.

8. Use cone-beam computed tomography (CBCT). This exposes the patient to a large amount of radiation (unless it is for some alternative reason) and is costly (Fig. 9.9).

Novel Use of Readily Available Materials to Locate the Screw Within a Cement-Retained Implant Restoration

What follows is a series of innovative and novel devices that are inexpensive and easily made. They can be fabricated either in the dental

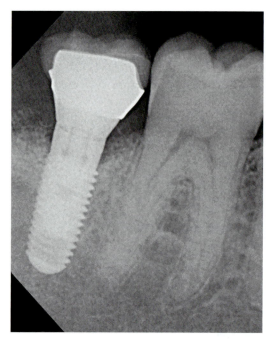

Fig. 9.4 Radiograph provides some information as to the long axis of the implant in the mesial-distal dimension but no indication of abutment form or position

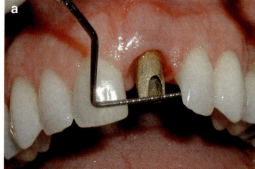

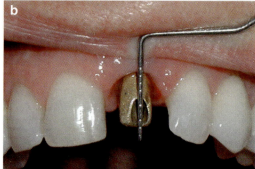

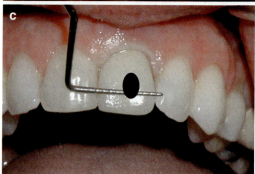

Fig. 9.6 (**a, b**) Pre-cementation photographic documentation of the site. When the crown is seated, the mark on the photograph (**c**) indicates the position of the screw access channel

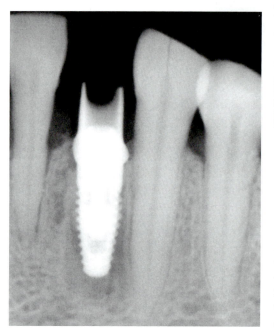

Fig. 9.5 Radiograph also gives information on the supporting abutment due to radiolucent ceramic crown

laboratory or chairside. The first described uses a paper clip, an implant screwdriver, and bite registration material. They offer many advantages over all other methods as being precise (they are true guides), easy to use, cheap, and can be readily modified if adjacent structures change.

Blu-Mousse® and Paper Clip

Step 1. Start with a sterilized paper clip and bend out an arm to assist holding the clip (Fig. 9.10).

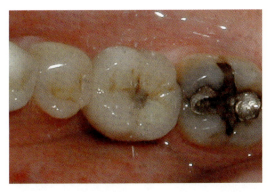

Fig. 9.7 A tattoo placed during fabrication marks the site of the screw channel. Patients may object; it has limited use in esthetic sites

Step 2. Use a new screw and an unworn driver that fits well within the screwhead. The screwdriver will then be a projection from the long axis of the screw (Fig. 9.11).

Step 3. Using the competed cast on which the implant restoration was made, remove the restoration but leave the abutment and abutment screw in place. Put the center of the paper clip over the abutment and hold it so it is elevated above the incisal edges of abutment and adjacent tooth sites. Index the adjacent tooth sites with registration material (Fig. 9.12). Blu-Mousse® fast-set (Parkell Inc, Edgewood, NY, USA) works well.

Step 4. Add more registration material to join the driver to the clip and surrounding registration material. *Note:* Do not add too much material in sites that would prevent the restoration from seating under the registration (Fig. 9.13).

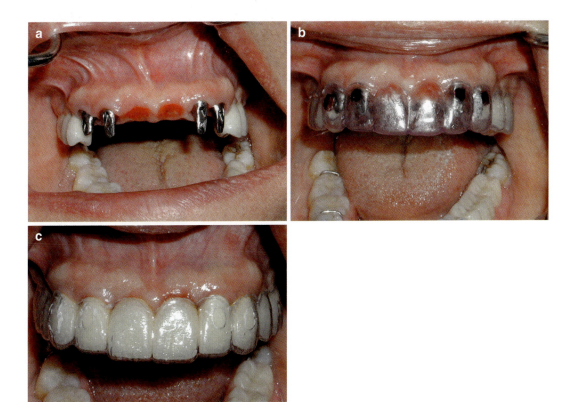

Fig. 9.8 (**a–c**) Vacuum-formed template is marked directly over the access hole site. These marks provide drill hole sites. Once transfered onto the restoration these sites relate to the abutment screw access hole beneath the restoration

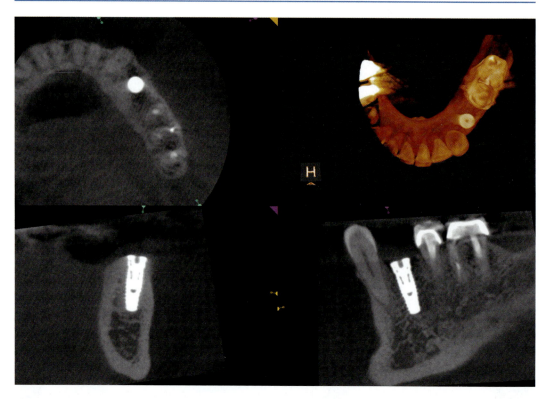

Fig. 9.9 A cone-beam computed image gives some indication of the angulation and position of the implant but still requires the clinician to "superimpose" this information by visual guessing

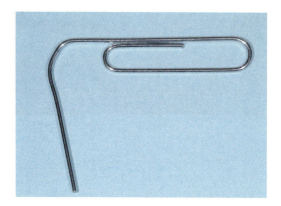

Fig. 9.10 Sterilized paper clip; one arm is bent out to act as a handle

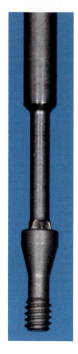

Step 5. Remove the index, remove the screwdriver, and clean up the embrasure areas so the index will reseat on the model with slight clearance once the crown is replaced (Fig. 9.14a, b).

Step 6. Store the index. If the screw does need to be accessed, place the index on site, and use the guide hole site and direction to plan the

Fig. 9.11 A screwdriver (Straumann) engages the head of an implant screw. Note how the shank of the screwdriver lies in the same long axial planes, acting as an extension of the screw

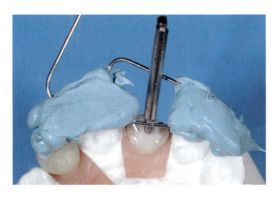

Fig. 9.12 The paper clip is centered on the implant abutment with the screwdriver projecting through it. The adjacent tooth sites have been indexed by using Blu-Mousse® (Parkell)

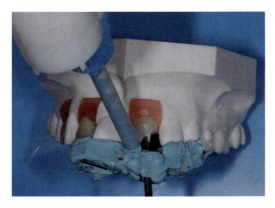

Fig. 9.13 Join the two adjacent tooth indexes and index the position of the screwdriver shank

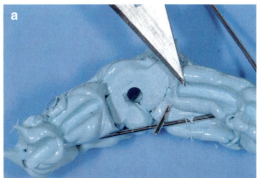

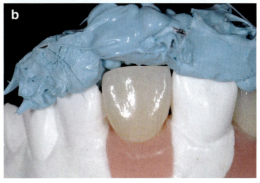

Fig. 9.14 (**a**) Remove material in the embrasure areas. This will allow the crown to be placed back on the model and the index should fit with space above the crown (**b**)

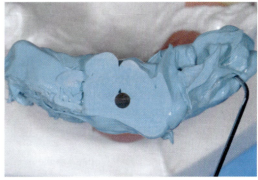

Fig. 9.15 From the occlusal view, the hole made by the screwdriver lies directly above the screwhead

drill hole (Fig. 9.15). *Note:* If the adjacent teeth change, then re-index them by removal of some registration material, then re-add to pick up the new index.

The Precision Implant Locator Device (PILD)

An improvement on this technique is to use a preformed device, the Precision Implant Locator Device (PILD). This consists of a preformed plate with a hole, the dimension of a latch-grip bur in its center. The hole enables a bur to be held at exactly 90° to the plate in the mesiodistal plane as well as the faciolingual plane.

With the help of a fast-setting vinylpolysiloxane (e.g., Blu-Mousse®), an implant screwdriver, and a simple plastic device, a directly located (site and angle and directional), minimal access channel resulting in the least possible damage can be made. The device acts as a three-dimensional guide or jig that has recorded the screw access channel site in the form of its trajectory.

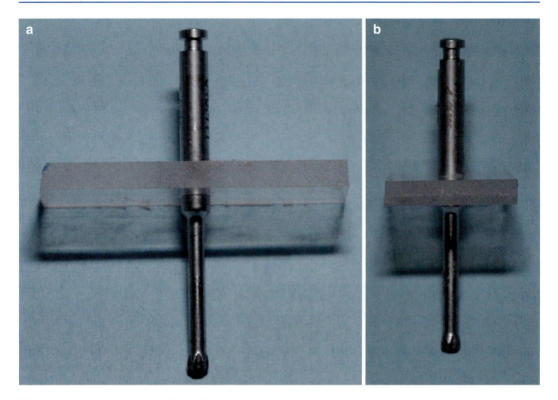

Fig. 9.16 (**a, b**) Plastic plate holding the latch-grip screwdriver at 90°

How to Make the Precision Implant Locator Device (PILD)

Step 1. Use a piece of flat, ridged plastic with dimensions about 25 mm long, 10 mm wide, and 3 mm thick.

Step 2. In the center of the plastic plate, prepare a hole 2.1 mm in diameter (this is the size of a latch-grip bur, used by most implant companies for the dimension of their screwdriver shanks). The hole must be perpendicular to the plate in all planes (Fig. 9.16a, b).

Step 3. On one side of the plate, make some retention pits or dimples using a bur. This will be the underside of the plate (Fig. 9.17).

Step 4. Place the appropriate screwdriver shank into the hole of the plate. *Note:* It should fit snuggly and project out at right angles to the plate. The screwdriver engaging side should project out from the underside. *Tip:* Unworn screwdrivers and new screws are essential for complete engagement.

Step 5. Place the screwdriver and plate assembly onto the implant model with just the implant

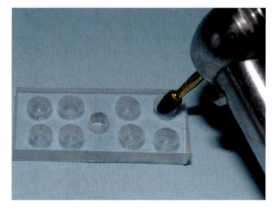

Fig. 9.17 Place retention dimples on one side of the plate—this becomes the "underside"

abutment in place. Engage the screw with the screwdriver and rotate the plate so it aligns and covers the adjacent sites that will be indexed. Ensure sufficient vertical space exists between all occlusal surfaces (about 0.5–1 mm) and the underside of the plate (Fig. 9.18).

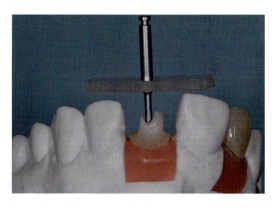

Fig. 9.18 PILD in place checking for position, not touching the model. The screwdriver has the same trajectory as the long axis of the implant

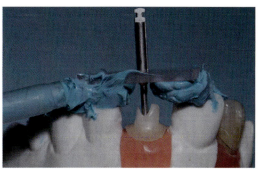

Fig. 9.20 PILD in use. The screwdriver is a trajectory of the implant long axis. Blu-Mousse® provides the indexing media for adjacent sites

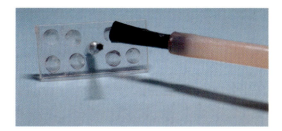

Fig. 9.19 PILD underside. Note retention dimples. Adhesive has been applied; screwdriver engages underside

Step 6. Apply polyvinyl siloxane adhesive agent onto the retention dimples on the underside of the PILD (Fig. 9.19).

Step 7. Apply Blu-Mousse® to either side of the screwdriver, directly onto the dimples. *Tip:* Use a slightly smaller extruder to control how much is expressed.

Step 8. Quickly seat onto the model, ensure the driver has locked itself correctly into the screwhead and allow to set (Fig. 9.20). *Tip:* When first trying this, use a longer setting time Blu-Mousse®.

Step 9. Remove the index, remove the screwdriver, and now try the PILD device to check that it is stable.

Step 10. Finally, make sure that the device will fit correctly when the restoration is put on the abutment (Fig. 9.21a). If not, clean the embrasure areas next to the crown, as the Blu-Mousse® may be preventing it from seating at this site. *Tip:* A sharp surgical blade does this nicely

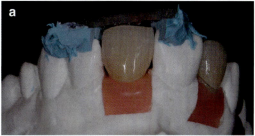

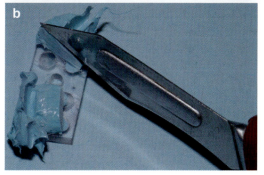

Fig. 9.21 (**a**) Check the PILD seats when the crown is in place on the model. It should not rock. (**b**) Cleaning the embrasures with a blade is usually necessary

(Fig. 9.21b). If you would like to make the PILD even more stable, add a little more Blu-Mousse® to the area of the crown (Fig. 9.22). Using a blade, carefully tidy the PILD (Fig. 9.23a, b). *Tip:* Do not block the trajectory hole.

Now the device is made and ready in case you ever need it (Figs. 9.24 and 9.25). Keep the PILD with the patient's records. It can also be used to record data on it, such as which implant was

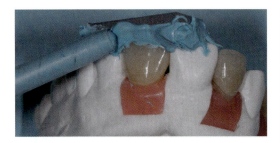

Fig. 9.22 Additional material may be added to stabilize the PILD if required but should not block the PILD hole

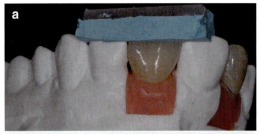

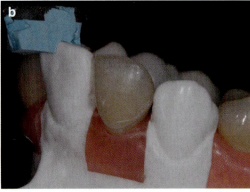

Fig. 9.23 (**a**, **b**) The PILD is cleaned up and checked to be stable. Buccal and lateral views of the guide in place on the model

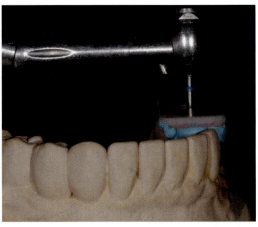

Fig. 9.25 A bur is placed in the PILD guide, and when held at 90° to the plate, it will give the site and direction of the underlying screw with minimal time and damage to the crown

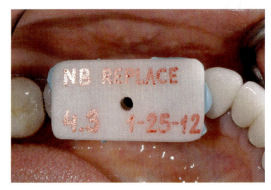

Fig. 9.26 Information can be stored on the PILD, including implant type, date, laboratory where it was fabricated, etc.

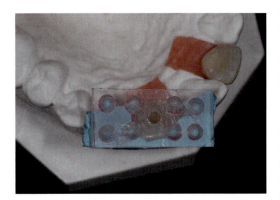

Fig. 9.24 Occlusal view of PILD guide (*Note:* Trajectory of the screw is visible)

used, the date, and laboratory (Fig. 9.26). The PILD can be given to the patients if they leave your office. Your laboratory can make these very easily for you. It provides a great service for our patients and may save you a lot of time, effort, and, yes, money in the future.

Should the restoration need to be removed and the screw accessed, place the device onto the site, hold the drill at 90° to the plate, and go! With Blu-Mousse®, there is the added advantage that should the indexing site change—for example, the restoration next to the implant is altered—then simply remove the Blu-Mousse® at that site, place the plate back on, and add some new Blu-Mousse®.

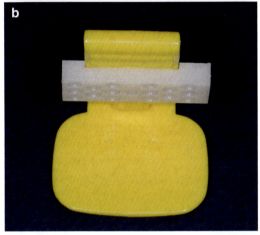

Fig. 9.27 (**a, b**) The PILD has now been adapted so it can also be used to connect to commercially available X-ray film and sensor holders. Recent studies have shown this method gives significantly more accurate information about bone levels and component fit

The PILD is currently being modified to enable it to be attached directly to commercial X-ray film holders. Because of its ability to record the long axis of the implant itself, and the plate lies 90° to this, with an attached X-ray holder, radiographs more accurately record component fit and bone levels (Fig. 9.27a, b).

Conclusion

Several techniques have been presented for locating the screw access channel of a cemented implant restoration. They vary in complexity and at which stage the record is made. Some are simple, requiring only a brief description of the screw access site prior to cementation, while others make use of cone-beam computed tomograms post-cementation.

It seems more prudent to accurately record the information prior to delivery of the final crown or bridge. Some devices can also provide information that the patients can keep with them if they move between clinics.

Bibliography

Daher T, Morgano SM. The use of digital photographs to locate implant abutment screws for implant-supported cement-retained restorations. J Prosthet Dent. 2008; 100:238–9.

Figueras-Alvarez O, Cedeño R, Cano-Batalla J, Cabratosa-Termes J. A method for registering the abutment screw position of cement-retained implant restorations. J Prosthet Dent. 2010;104(1):60–2.

Hill EE. A simple, permanent index for abutment screw access for cemented implant-supported crowns. J Prosthet Dent. 2007;97(5):313–4.

Lautensack J, Weber V, Wolfart S. Template to determine the position and angulation of the abutment screw channel for implant supported, cement retained restorations. J Prosthet Dent. 2012;107(2):134–6.

Lin K, Wadhwani C. A novel implant-locating device for abutment retrieval and making predictable radiographs to evaluate prosthetic misfit and health of osseointegration. Can J Res Dent. 2013;6:72–6.

Lin KC, Wadhwani CP, Sharma A, Finzen F. A radiograph positioning technique to evaluate prosthetic misfit and bone loss around implants. J Prosthet Dent. 2014a; 111(2):163–5.

Lin K, Wadhwani C, Sharma A, Finzen F, Cheng J. Assessing fit at the implant-abutment junction with a radiographic device that does not require access to the implant. J Prosthet Dent. 2014; 112(4):817–23.

Park JI, Yoon TH. A three-dimensional image-superimposition CAD/CAM technique to record the position and angulation of the implant abutment screw access channel. J Prosthet Dent. 2013;109:57–60.

Schwedhelm ER, Raigrodski A. A technique for locating implant abutment screws of posterior cement-retained metal-ceramic restorations with ceramic occlusal surfaces. J Prosthet Dent. 2006;95(2):165–7.

Tarica DY, Alvarado VM, Truong ST. Survey of United States dental schools on cementation protocols for implant crown restorations. J Prosthet Dent. 2010; 103(2):68–79.

Wadhwani C, Chung KH. Simple device for locating the abutment screw position of a cement-retained implant restoration. J Prosthet Dent. 2013;109:272–4.

Wicks R, Shintaku WH, Johnson A. Three-dimensional location of the retaining screw axis for a cemented single tooth implant restoration. J Prosthodont. 2012;21:491–3.

Intraoral Radiography and Implant Restoration

Chandur P.K. Wadhwani, Kevin C. Lin,
and Curtis S.K. Chen

Abstract

One of the most useful tools available for implant dentistry is radiography, from initial assessment all the way through to long-term health monitoring of the peri-implant tissues. The restorative dentist frequently uses intraoral radiography to conduct evaluations on implant component fit and the bone related to the implant. However, limitations exist arising from the way radiographs are made as well as how they are interpreted. Clinically significant factors will be discussed in this chapter, as well as ways to improve the diagnostic value of intraoral radiographs.

Introduction

The planning and surgical phases of implant dentistry often involve modern, sophisticated three-dimensional imaging equipment and techniques, which few dental offices currently possess. This

C.P.K. Wadhwani, BDS, MSD (✉)
Department of Restorative Dentistry,
University of Washington, Seattle, WA, USA

Private Practice Limited to Prosthodontics,
1200, 116th Ave NE #A, Bellevue, WA 98004, USA
e-mail: cpkw@uw.edu

K.C. Lin, DDS
Department of Integrated Reconstructive Dental
Sciences, University of the Pacific, Arthur A. Dugoni
School of Dentistry, San Francisco, CA, USA

C.S.K. Chen, DDS, MSD, PhD
Department of Oral Medicine,
University of Washington School of Dentistry,
Seattle, WA 98195, USA
e-mail: cskchen@uw.edu

is in contrast to the implant restorative and follow-up phases, where more traditional two-dimensional intraoral radiography (IOR) is more commonly used as a diagnostic tool, with the equipment necessary readily available in most dental offices. When used appropriately, IOR can provide clinically relevant information in a minimally invasive, inexpensive, and immediate manner. It remains the preferred method for most clinicians when evaluating hard dental tissues, especially bone where implants are involved.

Intraoral Radiography: Uses and Limitations

Intraoral radiography (IOR) has been useful for the detection of pathology, visualization of trabecular bone pattern, and highlighting of anatomical aberrations and adjacent tooth angulations that may affect the restoration path

C.P.K. Wadhwani (ed.), *Cementation in Dental Implantology: An Evidence-Based Guide*,
DOI 10.1007/978-3-642-55163-5_10, © Springer-Verlag Berlin Heidelberg 2015

163

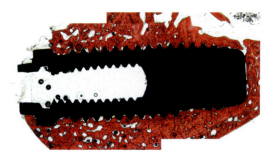

Fig. 10.1 Histological section of an osseointegrated implant. The red part is the bone; the black item is the implant. Notice the tight adaptation of bone to the implant. Thirty-five percent to 40 % of the mineralized content is in contact with the implant surface

of insertion. It can also offer useful information with respect to the mechanical alignment and union of the implant components, which is considered vital for the long-term success of the implant restoration. Radiographs have also been used to evaluate the success of dental implants as well as to provide a means of monitoring their long-term health. This is accomplished by comparing successive images to baseline records over a period of time.

However, as with any diagnostic test, limitations exist. Some are the result of the radiographic processes in general; others have to do with the technique-sensitive nature of the equipment and making the radiographic image. Also, the diagnostic value of any given radiograph varies, depending upon the pathological process being examined, as well as the ability or expertise of the clinician evaluating the radiographic image. It is also known that IOR can give false negatives; in other words, a disease process or issue may present but may not be detected, especially in the early pathological and/or bone remodeling phase (Fig. 10.1). Given this information, the prudent clinician will use IOR as part of the evaluation process along with other clinical assessment methods. Specifically with implant therapy, IOR can supplement the clinical implant site examination along with other signs, for example, inflammation, recession, probing pocket depth, and mobility. Consistent with all radiographic examinations, IOR should be applied according to a strategy to reduce patient exposure to radiation. The radiograph should be made and developed to be of

the highest quality possible to provide as much information as possible to the clinician.

Even given these limitations, IOR still provides some degree of quantitative and qualitative analysis that may be extremely useful. The purpose of this chapter is to evaluate and give guidance to the clinician regarding the appropriate use of IOR, specifically during the restorative phases of implant therapy and subsequent monitoring and follow-up.

IOR, Bone-to-Implant Contact and Health of the Tissues

Implant dentistry frequently focuses on the bone directly adjacent to the implant. In fact, osseointegration is defined as "the apparent direct attachment or connection of osseous tissue to an inert, alloplastic material without intervening connective tissue." Although radiographic assessments of bone adjacent to the dental implant are made, it should be understood that direct implant–bone contact cannot be accurately determined. Because IOR is two-dimensional, there exists an inability to discern bone levels directly facial and lingual to the implant body, as these sites will be obscured by the implant itself. Even at interproximal sites adjacent to the implant, bone attachment cannot be easily determined.

A study on the accuracy of radiographs to diagnose radiolucencies surrounding implants was undertaken by Sewerin. A series of implants were inserted into bone, some with intimate contact to bone, while others had an intentional gap of varying size created between the implant and the socket. These were radiographed under standardized conditions and then evaluated by 10 experienced implant clinicians who were asked to judge the likelihood that a space was present. The inter-observer agreement was low and the diagnostic accuracy was greatest only when a 0.175 mm space existed. It was concluded that, in general, radiographs were an unreliable method for diagnosing peri-implant spaces. However, their value improved with increasing space widths up to 175 μm between the implant and surrounding bone. Clinically, the study has implications in that radiology cannot be relied on as the only means of determining the extent of bone to implant contact.

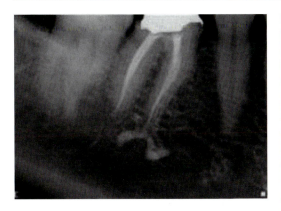

Fig. 10.2 An example of alveolar space. The endodontist has used calcium hydroxide as an interim treatment. During the process of placing this into the root canal system, some has been extruded. Note the radiopacity in areas of the alveolar spaces that were previously occupied by marrow space

Bone-to-implant contact is the amount of bone that generally contacts the implant body. Bone is composed of both mineralized and non-mineralized material of varying degree and is in large part dependent upon the type or character of bone being examined. This results in the actual mineralized bone contact often being limited to only 35–40 % of the implant surface, as seen in Fig. 10.1, which further compounds the ability to determine how much bone is truly in contact with an implant when relying on IOR.

Implants are generally placed into cancellous or alveolar bone. The word alveolar is derived from the Latin "alveolus" meaning "little cavity." Therefore, this bone is not solid, but rather consists of many little cavities within it. The alveolar or marrow spaces, which are filled with readily displaced non-mineralized tissue, can frequently be highlighted by endodontic processes (Fig. 10.2) with the intrusion of radiopaque material.

The ability to assess the status of implants at any stage is important, and apart from routine monitoring it should be considered a prerequisite to know and record the health status prior to reconstruction, at the commencement of a restoration, or when a replacement prosthesis is being considered. Radiographs can also provide a baseline standard against which subsequent radiographs can be compared to monitor changes

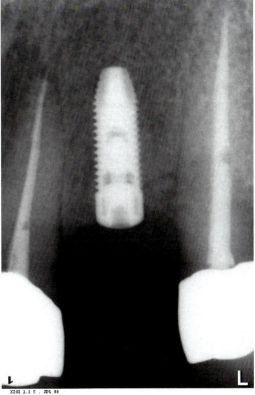

Fig. 10.3 This radiograph was made prior to the commencement of the final restoration. It provides some information about possible pathological issues, the type of bone, how deep the implant is placed, and potential angulation issues with adjacent teeth. It can also be used as a reference to compare future serial radiographs against to evaluate long-term changes, provided they are all standardized

over time, provided there is adherence to some form of standardization (Fig. 10.3).

Marginal bone height around implants has been used as a measure for monitoring bone health. Again, in vitro studies have reported on potential errors, suggesting in clinical cases distortion of buccal and lingual bone margins may result in an overestimation of bone heights. The degree of overestimation is influenced by the buccolingual position of the implant. Again, even given these limitations, it is advised that a baseline record should be made with an exacting technique that controls for factors such as position and angulation relative to the implant position prior to the fabrication of a new or replacement restoration.

Mechanical Connection of Implant Components

Visual examination may be possible if the implant head connection to the impression coping is above or very near the free gingival margin. If not, tactile perception may be considered, but a radiograph made with the correct angulation may provide the most useful data.

Periapical radiographs can be a useful adjunct to determine the accuracy of fit for a prosthesis. They provide high-dimensional accuracy, image detail, and minimal magnification and distortion when they are made correctly. To utilize the advantage of intraoral radiography, it is absolutely critical to maintain the X-ray beam perpendicular to the implant's component connection junction (CCJ). The component connection can be at the crown–abutment junction or abutment–fixture junction. When the proper long-cone paralleling technique is adopted, they offer significant diagnostic value for the dentists and minimal negative health impact on the patients. Inadequate fit of components may result in failure of the prosthesis and the retaining screws connecting the implants to the superstructure and may also have the potential to cause implant-to-bone changes (Fig. 10.4).

Proper radiographs can help clinicians evaluate the fit at the CCJ, but improper alignment between the fixture and the X-ray beam could result in not detecting a misfit and mislead clinicians about the true fit of the implant components. Radiographically detectable edges of the abutment and head of fixture become smaller as the divergence of the X-ray beam increases. Laboratory studies have also confirmed that as the angulation of the X-ray tube diverges away from the angle perpendicular to a restorative margin or the long axis of the implant fixture, identifying misfit becomes increasingly difficult. A model was fabricated with an implant and a spacer providing a gap of 100 μm with the healing cap. Radiographs were made at 0° (orthogonal), 10°, 20°, and 30°. The radiographs produced are seen in Fig. 10.5a–g.

The angulation of the X-ray tube head relative to the implant long axis is critical. Under

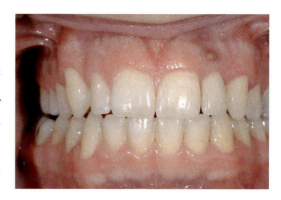

Fig. 10.4 The restoration was placed on an implant, which trapped tissue between the implant body and abutment (CCJ). Once the tissue was released, the inflammation resolved. Follow-up revealed no further lesions

optimum conditions, gaps of 0.05 mm may be detectable, but become obscured when deviations of the X-ray tube head are 5° or more to the long axis of the implant. Gaps of 0.1 mm or larger can also be detected with 10–15° X-ray beam incidence away from the long axis. However, when the incident beam is greater than 10–15°, as seen in Fig. 10.5e, f, these gaps also become obscured. Other factors that also alter the ability to detect gaps include radiographic focal spot size and Focus film distance (FFD). This is the distance between the X-ray source and the film or sensor receptor in diagnostic radiography.

If the goal of treatment is to determine exacting component fit, then clearly the tube angulation must be strictly controlled. This becomes more of a challenge when restorations are splined (Fig. 10.6a, b). The fit of a splinted restoration on implants or a fixed partial denture may present with particular issues related to non-passive fit. Laboratory processes, along with embedment relaxation effects that occur when metal components are connected with screw joints, make multiple implant connection particularly susceptible to non-passive fit errors. When evaluating the seating of such a prosthesis, the individual implant positions must be accounted for with each attachment site (Fig. 10.7a, b).

It is clear that in evaluating for the fit of implant components, the radiographic image is subject to distortions as a result of angulation

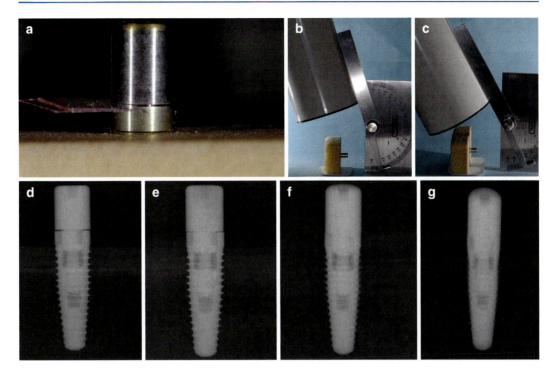

Fig. 10.5 (**a–g**) These radiographs were made by altering the X-ray cone relative to the implant and healing abutment by (**d**) 0°, (**e**)10°, (**f**) 20°, and (**g**) 30°. They show how minor errors in angulation alter the ability to detect component fit

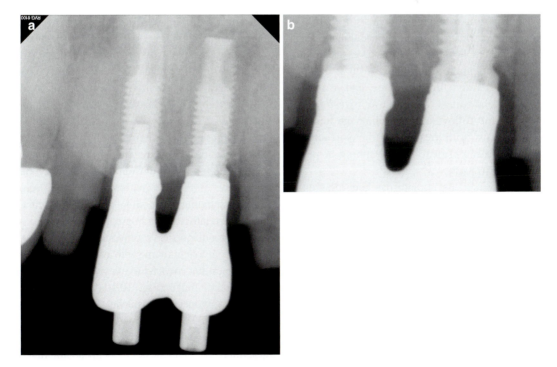

Fig. 10.6 (**a, b**) Radiograph at metal try-in appointment. Enlarged image shows intimate contact of both abutments with the implants

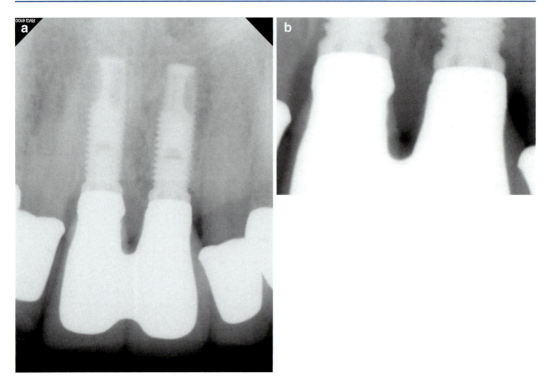

Fig. 10.7 (**a, b**) On final delivery, an orthogonal radiograph indicates a misfit on the left central implant. The prosthesis was remade

effects. Several studies have evaluated these artifacts and how they develop, assessing the relative angulations of X-ray tube, implant body angle, and film or image sensor angulation. The findings from these investigations suggest the following: determine the angle of the implant with respect to the surrounding occlusal plane prior to radiographing, if possible (Fig. 10.8a, b).

However, if the implant has been previously restored, it may be more difficult to determine the orientation without first removing the restoration. The angulation of the X-ray tube head relative to the implant long axis is critical. If the goal of treatment is to determine exacting component fit, then clearly the tube angulation must be strictly controlled. In the horizontal plane, if the incident X-rays are perpendicular to the long axis of the implant (orthogonal), the mesial and distal tube head angulations are not critical as long as the gap size is uniform; it will be detected from any angle. As a result of this information it is sug-

gested that, given a knowledge of the implant angulation, the tube head orientation in the vertical plane is most critical. To standardize sequential radiographs, a paralleling device may be of use, for example, RINN systems (Dentsply Rinn, Elgin, IL USA). However, the holder should be oriented relative to the implant long axis rather than the occlusal surfaces, which more commonly occurs and produces information that may be inaccurate.

Understanding the component structures and how these relate to the radiographic images seen is also vital for diagnosis of component fit (Fig. 10.9). Implant components come with a variety of matching surfaces that can lead to misinterpretation of a radiographic image (Fig. 10.10a, b). When an implant component only touches at the periphery, a radiographic anomaly known as the "peripheral eggshell effect" may result. This may lead to the false impression that the components do not match or have failed. This would be an incorrect assumption.

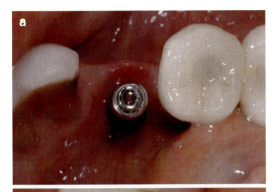

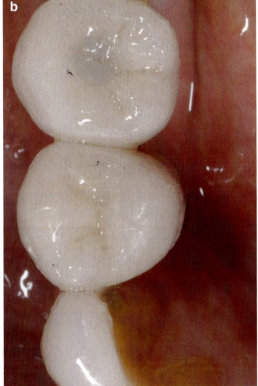

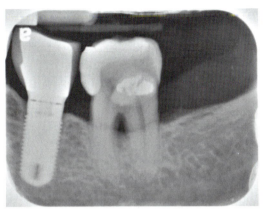

Fig. 10.9 Understanding the radiographic properties of the implant system, it appears as if this Zimmer AdVent implant abutment only seats onto the implant body mesially and distally. This is a radiographic artifact—the so-called peripheral eggshell effect (PESE)

Fig. 10.8 (**a**) It is important to access the implant with respect to radiographic techniques. This implant is angled toward the midline, which must be taken into account when making radiographs. (**b**) Now restored, the underlying implant's orientation can only be guessed at

The Value of Orthogonal Radiography with Implants: Connection and Health

For determining implant component fit, there are ways to provide for orthogonal radiographs to be made. To ensure a perpendicular relationship

between the X-ray beam and the implant components, all existing paralleling devices usually attach directly to the implant body at the time of making radiographs. This is a limiting factor because the implant restoration would have to be deconstructed for access to the implant itself; therefore, radiographic assessments can generally only be done on screw-retained restorations or implant bars where the implant access channel is not permanently blocked (Fig. 10.11). In addition, by having to deconstruct the implant prosthesis, the paralleling devices may disrupt the peri-implant tissues and affect their overall health, thus limiting the capacity to monitor crestal bone loss. So, in reality, component misfit can only be evaluated.

By indexing the implant fixture to the adjacent dentition or anatomical landmark, the authors developed a novel X-ray paralleling device, the Precision Implant X-ray Relator and Locator (PIXRL), that can be attached to commercially available film holders. The PIXRL is first positioned perpendicularly to the implant fixture using implant drivers or implant placement drivers; it then allows for registration record to be made between the adjacent teeth or anatomical landmark and the positioned PIXRL jig. The sequence is described in greater detail with the provided illustrations (Fig. 10.12a–e). Because the occlusal relationship is indexed with the adja-

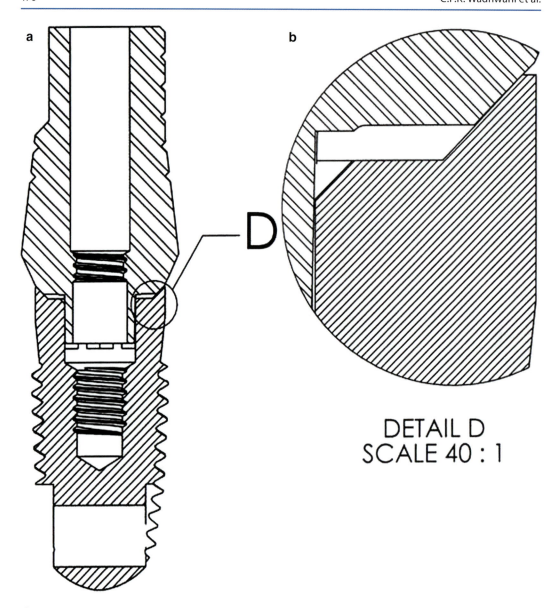

Fig. 10.10 (**a**) The PESE results from the margin of the abutment contacting the lip of the implant only. (**b**) Enlarged image. This must be understood; failure would result in potential misdiagnosis of the components not fitting together correctly (Reprinted with permission by Dentistry Today Wahdwani (2012). Intraoral Radiography and Dental Implant Restoration. Dent Today August 2013; Vol. 31; 8:70])

cent teeth, accurate radiographs can be made consistently without the removal of implant prosthesis thereafter; the evaluation of CCJ occurs at the abutment level.

A study was conducted at the University of California, San Francisco, to compare whether misfit at the AFJ can be more accurately and confidently assessed using radiographs made with the PIXRL X-ray paralleling device in a clinically simulated model. A microgap ranging from 0, 50, to 100 μm was introduced at the AFJ of a provisional implant crown in a manikin-typodont

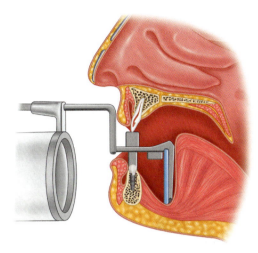

Fig. 10.11 Example of existing devices that allow true orthogonal standard X-rays to be made. All must attach to the implant body (fixture) directly at each and during X-ray exposure (Reprinted from Cox and Pharoah (1986). Copyright © 1986, with permission from Elsevier)

assembly (Fig. 10.13a–c). In 50 and 100 μm misfit conditions where PIXRL was used, clinicians were able to detect prosthetic misfit with 77.8 and 100 % accuracy, respectively. Without the use of PIXRL, clinicians were able to detect only 16.1 % of the misfit in 50 μm gap and 92.6 % of the misfit in 100 μm gap. The sample of radiographs made under each misfit condition (0 um, 50 um, 100 um) is provided (Fig. 10.14a–f). Consistent with previous findings, the study effectively demonstrated that paralleling devices are critical in helping clinicians obtain diagnostic radiographs for implant assessment. How the device provides orthogonal radiographs is demonstrated in Fig. 10.15a, b.

Limitation with Radiography and Professional Responsibility

Adopting the use of a paralleling device in making clinical radiographs provides an opportunity for clinicians to monitor changes in bone architecture or prosthetic misfit around an implant accurately and consistently over time.

Anatomical limitations (i.e., missing teeth, the palatal vault contour, shallow lingual sulcus, presence of tori, or unfavorable mandibular arch form) and patient factors (i.e., prominent gag reflex or psychological issues) may restrict the use of such devices. The application of the device in various clinical situations must also be considered.

The accuracy of an intraoral radiograph inevitably reduces the number of X-ray images to be remade in a clinical situation; if the clinician can be more certain about the diagnostic quality of a radiograph, there would be less need for exposing patients to additional radiation. Claus and colleagues have recently correlated dental X-rays to an increased risk of meningioma in a population-based case–control study. Despite the shortcomings in its study design, the subsequent negative publicity generated reminded the entire dental community of the significance of minimizing the patient's radiation exposure when possible.

Intraoral radiography, although considered somewhat basic, has certain advantages over more sophisticated radiographic examinations from cone beam computer tomography and panoramic radiography, as listed below.

Cone Beam CT
1. 'Sunburst' effect due to x-ray scattering from metallic components may make detecting misfit challenging
2. Limited resolution (local cone beam has highest resolution at 70um)
3. Expensive

Panoral Radiograph
1. High false negative rate in detecting small gaps due to inherent limitations such as magnification, distortion, negative vertical angulation of projection, and patient movement
2. Limited resolution

A protocol should be developed by the clinician to determine when radiographs should be made. This is especially important during the initial pick-up impression, seating of the final

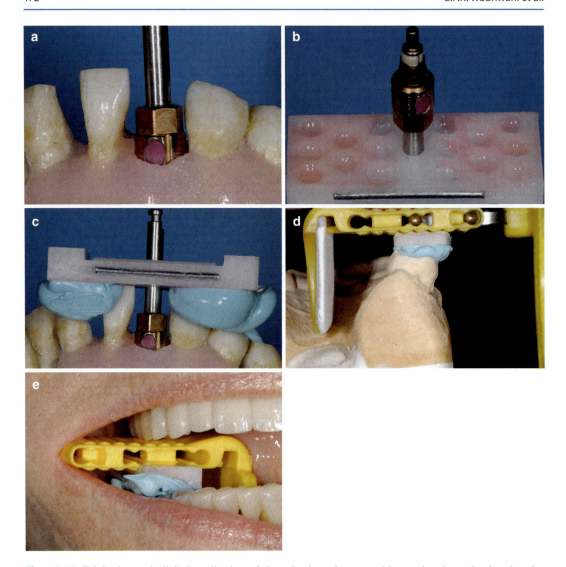

Fig. 10.12 Fabrication and clinical application of the X-ray paralleling device are critical in helping operators obtain diagnostic radiographs for implant assessment. (**a**) Access to implant fixture obtained intraorally or from implant master cast; implant placement driver is attached to the fixture. (**b**) Connect the paralleling PIXRL device to shank of implant placement driver; adhesive is applied on undersurface of the jig. (**c**) Orient PIXRL jig assembly to implant placement driver and make occlusal registration record against adjacent teeth. (**d**) Attach radiographic film holder to PIXRL jig; use occlusal registration record to maintain orientation of film holder and radiographic film. (**e**) Adopt conventional parallel-cone technique to make radiographs intraorally with device (film holder paralleling arm was attached for actual clinical use; it was only removed here for better visualization of PIXRL assembly)

abutment, completion of the restoration, and any other clinical situations when the component fit cannot be directly verified by sight or feel. When a restoration is to be cemented onto an implant abutment and where a connection is not accessible, for example, when it lies beneath the peri-implant tissues, it would be prudent to radiograph the components before final cementation to confirm they match as intended. This is to confirm that the abutment is correctly

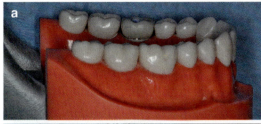
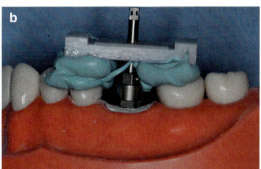
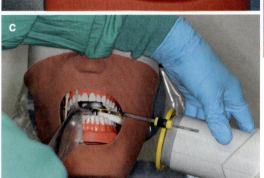

Fig. 10.13 The simulated clinical study. (**a**) The implant crown was fabricated with proper anatomy and occlusion by building composite on the modified UCLA abutment. (**b**) The PIXRL jig is indexed to the implant fixture and the adjacent dentition using an implant placement driver and a vinyl polysiloxane bite registration material. (**c**) The assistants were asked to position X-ray film holding assembly and the X-ray tube in a routine manner. They were free to use cotton roll, gauze, or cotton pad as they saw necessary

located onto the implant, as well as to confirm that the crown seats onto the abutment itself. Failure to do so may fail to detect errors as a result of fabrication, or components not seating (Fig. 10.16).

Cemented Implant Restorations

There is increasing evidence that residual excess cement may lead to peri-implant disease. It is the responsibility of the implant-restoring dentist to ensure and check that no excess cement invades and remains in the peri-implant tissues. One way of confirming that excess has been removed is by the use of IOR. However, there is no standard for the radiopacity required of implant cements, which is problematic. An in vitro study and case studies have reported on the ability to detect commonly used implant cements radiographically. The results indicated that many cements would not be easily found, and some not at all, at any given thickness, as shown earlier in Fig. 10.14a–c. While there is no ideal implant cement, the onus must be on the restoring clinician to choose one that can be readily seen radiographically and to understand the characteristics of the cement extrusion patterns that may present with IOR. When a radiopaque cement is used, a radiograph may be used to determine if residual excess cement exists (see Fig. 10.15a).

Implant Health and Follow-Up

Much has been written about the success of dental implants, with radiographic evaluation used for

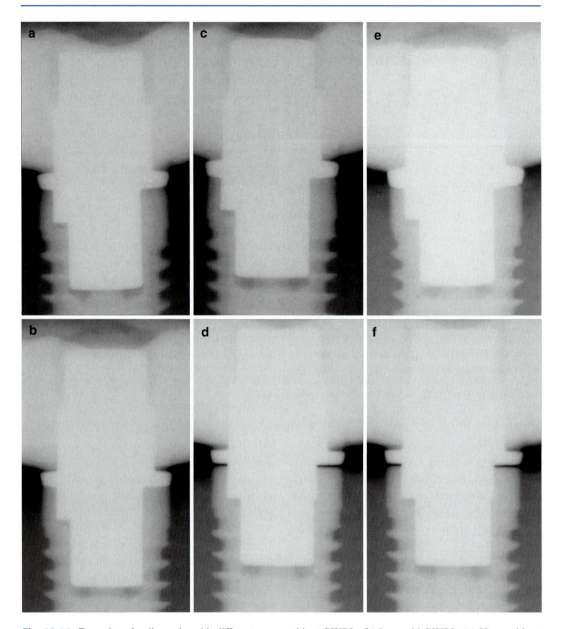

Fig. 10.14 Examples of radiographs with different gap dimension, from 0 to 100 μm, typical of those produced in the study with and without the PIXRL device. (**a**) 0 μm without PIXRL; (**b**) 0 μm with PIXRL; (**c**) 50 μm without PIXRL; (**d**) 50 μm with PIXRL; (**e**) 100 μm without PIXRL; (**f**) 100 μm with PIXRL

measurements. The early criteria for implant success included values related to acceptable bone loss and time. IOR has been used as a tool to evaluate hard tissue health, but again, there are limitations with this method of assessment. Mineral loss from bone is not consistently or easily quantified and varies from site to site. The difference lies in the initial mineral content, the alveolar content, and the amount of cortical bone in the area evaluated. Early studies suggested that mineral loss needed to exceed 7 % of the mass before it may be detected on a film radiograph in the maxilla, but mineral loss in the mandible may have to be as great as 30 % before it is readily detected. More

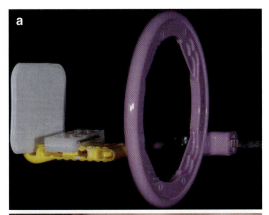

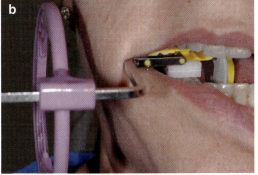

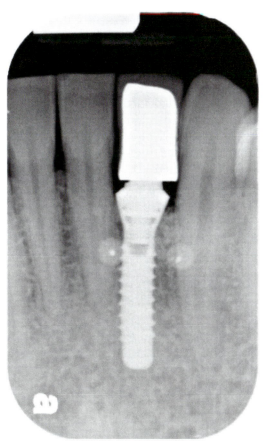

Fig. 10.15 (**a**, **b**) How the PIXRL attaches to a paralleling device. Once the PIXRL is indexed to the implant, consistent standardized radiographs are possible to monitor bone health as well as confirm connection of the abutment

Fig. 10.16 This restoration was cemented onto the abutment. No pre-cementation radiograph was made; the crown did not seat as intended. It is likely the adjacent teeth contacted the restoration prematurely, preventing its placement. The restoring dentist failed to detect this error

recent studies have reported on mineral loss as a result of osteoporosis and have suggested that detectable mineral changes may be as little as 1.2 % with photo-stimulable phosphor systems.

Frequently, studies compare marginal bone loss measurements; however this may be problematic. Marginal bone height adjacent to implants is highly susceptible to angulation effects relative to X-ray film and implant (see Fig. 10.15a). The ability to obtain consistent perpendicular radiographs that will provide diagnostic relevance is problematic. Devices exist that are directly screwed into the implant body itself that allow the film, X-ray tube, and implant body axis to be related. However, once the implant restoration is placed, this becomes impractical, as removal of the restoration at subsequent visits is both time consuming and may alter the soft tissues and bone levels around the

implant, as it is known that the disruption caused by removal and replacement of the abutment may lead to loss of the implant supporting tissues. One means of standardizing IOR is to develop more practical devices that align the implant body to the X-ray beam precisely, but do not require the removal of the restoration on subsequent visits.

To date, few protocols have been developed that recommend specific time intervals for radiographic evaluation. However, data from one study suggests a correlation between probing attachment levels and radiographic presentation. It was noted that probing attachment levels obtained with a periodontal probe at 1, 3, and 6 months after loading proved to be a good indicator of peri-implant radiographic status at 2 years. Conversely, radiographically assessed tissue changes observed during the same test periods of 1, 3, and 6 months were good indicators of probing attachment levels expected at 2 years. This relationship between probing and radiographic evaluation may be used to assess examination needs, suggesting that when changes in probing levels occur, radiographic assessment may be advised. For longitudinal research purposes, it is recommended that radiographs be obtained at baseline, 1 year, 3 years, and 5 years, and thereafter every 5 years. How this relates to everyday clinical practice procedures has yet to be ascertained.

Conclusion

The usefulness of intraoral radiography has been described, along with its limitations when considering implant restorations. One major issue is the alignment of the incident X-rays so that they are consistently perpendicular to the implant body, to provide the most reliable information possible. Other limitations include inconsistencies as a result of the inability to verify the nature and extent of bone around an implant, which is subject to variation as a result of type of bone and site. Where implants are concerned, as a diagnostic tool, IOR should be considered as part of a multitude of tests—including probing, mobility, symptoms, and other soft tissue evaluations. It must be emphasized that IOR cannot be relied upon as being the sole diagnostic test.

Bibliography

Abrahamsson I, Berglundh T, Lindhe J. The mucosal barrier following abutment dis/reconnection. An experimental study in dogs. J Clin Periodontol. 1997;24:568–72.

Albrektsson T, Zarb G, Worthington P, Eriksson AR. The longterm efficacy of currently used dental implants: a review and proposed criteria of success. Int J Oral Maxillofac Implants. 1986;1:11–25.

Begoña Ormaechea M, Millstein P, Hirayama H. Tube angulation effect on radiographic analysis of the implant-abutment interface. Int J Oral Maxillofac Implants. 1999;14:77–85.

Bender IB. Factors influencing the radiographic appearance of bony lesions. J Endod. 1997;23:5–14.

Benn DK. Estimating the validity of radiographic measurements of marginal bone height changes around osseointegrated implants. Implant Dent. 1992;1:79–83.

Brägger U. Use of radiographs in evaluating success, stability and failure in implant dentistry. Periodontol 2000. 1998;17:77–88.

Cameron SM, Joyce A, Brousseau JS, Parker MH. Radiographic verification of implant abutment seating. J Prosthet Dent. 1998;79:298–303.

Couture RA, Whiting BR, Hildebolt CF, Dixon DA. Visibility of trabecular structures in oral radiographs. Oral Surg Oral Med Oral Pathol Oral Radiol Endod. 2003;96:764–71.

Cox JF, Pharoah M. An alternative holder for radiographic evaluation of tissue-integrated prostheses. J Prosthet Dent. 1986;56:338–41.

Lin KC, Wadhwani CP, Sharma A, Finzen F. A radiograph positioning technique to evaluate prosthetic misfit and bone loss around implants. J Prosthet Dent. 2014;111(2):163–5.

Meijer HJ, Steen WH, Bosman F. Standardized radiographs of the alveolar crest around implants in the mandible. J Prosthet Dent. 1992;68:318–21.

Misch CE. Dental implant prosthetics. St. Louis: Mosby Elsevier; 2005.

Regan JE, Mitchell DF. Evaluation of periapical radiolucencies found in cadavers. J Am Dent Assoc. 1963;66:529–33.

Salvi GE, Lang NP. Diagnostic parameters for monitoring peri-implant conditions. Int J Oral Maxillofac Implants. 2004;19(suppl):116–27.

Sewerin IP. Radiographic control of fixture-abutment connection in Brånemark implant technique. Scand J Dent Res. 1989;97:559–64.

Sewerin IP. Errors in radiographic assessment of marginal bone height around osseointegrated implants. Scand J Dent Res. 1990;98:428–33.

Sewerin IP, Gotfredsen K, Stoltze K. Accuracy of radiographic diagnosis of peri-implant radiolucencies—an in vitro experiment. Clin Oral Implants Res. 1997;8:299–304.

The glossary of prosthodontic terms. J Prosthet Dent. 2005;94:10–92.

Trisi P, Lazzara R, Rebaudi A, Rao W, Testori T, Porter SS. Bone-implant contact on machined and dual acid-etched surfaces after 2 months of healing in the human maxilla. J Periodontol. 2003;74:945–56.

Wadhwani C, Hess T, Faber T, Piñeyro A, Chen CS. A descriptive study of the radiographic density of implant restorative cements. J Prosthet Dent. 2010;103:295–302.

Wadhwani C, Rapoport D, La Rosa S, Hess T, Kretschmar SD. Radiographic detection and characteristic patterns of residual excess cement associated with cement-retained implant restorations: a clinical report. J Prosthet Dent. 2012a;107:151–7.

Wadhwani CP, Schuler R, Taylor S, Chen CS. Intraoral radiography and dental implant restoration. Dent Today. 2012b;31(8):66, 68, 70–1.

White SC, Pharoah MJ. Oral radiology: principles and interpretation. 6th ed. St. Louis: Mosby Elsevier; 2009.

Treatment Options Related to Cement Contamination and Repair of Lesions

11

Ken M. Akimoto and Ralf F. Schuler

Abstract

Periodic evaluation of the implant and restoration should be made to monitor overall health. The examination should include mobility (restoration as well as implant), probing (depth and especially bleeding on probing), plaque score, radiographic and visual tissue examination (color, texture, tissue dimension changes), recession, and suppuration. The ability for the patient to adequately clean and maintain the implant site is also vitally important, and this too should be assessed regularly. The level of therapy required to restore implant health will be determined by the severity of the issue, which can often be determined during these examinations. Sequential information and how this changes between examinations will also give an indication of progression, although it must be remembered that peri-implant disease may have a unique pattern of onset time and progression, very different from periodontal disease.

Introduction

Dental implants can predictably achieve osseointegration and retain implant-supported restorations in function with long-term success. Failures of dental implants, however, are a clinical reality, and implant-related complications can be attributed to many factors including, but not limited to, surgical complications, prosthetic or mechanical failures, and biological complications. Biological complications consist of adverse changes in the peri-implant support, presenting mainly as inflammation and peri-implant bone loss (Fig. 11.1). The ultimate, tangible end point of biological complications might be the loss of the dental implant subsequent to persistent inflammatory changes in the surrounding mucosal tissues and/or progressive peri-implant bone loss.

This chapter will illuminate the potential role of residual excess cement as an etiologic factor for the development of biological complications around dental implants. The importance of a

K.M. Akimoto, DDS, MSD (✉)
Department of Periodontics, University of Washington, Private Practice Limited to Periodontics and Implant, Issaquah, WA, USA

Department of Periodontics, University of Washington School of Dentistry, Seattle, WA, USA
e-mail: ken@nwperio.com

R.F. Schuler, Dr. Med. Dent, MSD
Department of Periodontics, University of Washington School of Dentistry, Seattle, WA, USA

Department of Periodontics, Private Practice Limited to Periodontics and Implant Dentistry, Seattle, WA, USA

C.P.K. Wadhwani (ed.), *Cementation in Dental Implantology: An Evidence-Based Guide*,
DOI 10.1007/978-3-642-55163-5_11, © Springer-Verlag Berlin Heidelberg 2015

thorough clinical examination and diagnostic radiographs will be demonstrated, and potential treatment options will be discussed.

Clinical Examination

Periodic post-treatment examination of dental implants is of utmost importance since implant complications can often be treated successfully when detected early. Without periodic re-examinations, peri-implant disease might not be detected early enough due to the absence of tangible clinical symptoms. The American Academy of Periodontology issued a paper in 2003 on periodontal maintenance stating, "patients should be evaluated at regular intervals to monitor their peri-implant status, the condition of the

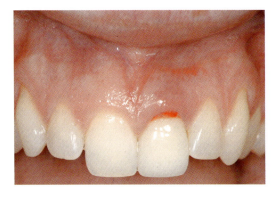

Fig. 11.1 Clinical example of a dental implant (maxillary left central incisor) exhibiting biological complications following restoration

implant supported prostheses, and plaque control." Some authorities recommend regular peri-implant re-evaluations every 3 months during the first year after restoration, followed by less frequent office visits thereafter. Evaluation of the dental implant includes but is not necessarily limited to radiographic examination, implant stability tests, analysis of microbial profiles, peri-implant probing, and assessment of clinical attachment levels.

Diagnostic periapical and vertical bitewing radiographs should be taken at the time of implant placement to establish baseline bone levels and at the time of delivery of the final implant-supported restoration. Subsequent radiographs should be ordered as indicated and compared to the baseline to rule out progressive peri-implant bone loss (<0.1 mm bone remodeling per year, 1 year after implant placement).

Implant stability measurements using impact resistance (Periotest, Avtec Dental, Mount Pleasant, SC, USA) or resonance frequency analysis (RFA) could be implemented during post-treatment. Automated implant stability meters are readily available that measure the implant stability quotient (ISQ) value as an indicator for the level of osseointegration in dental implants. The ISQ scale ranges from 1 to 100, and values from 55 to 85 indicate acceptable stability ranges. The cause of any implant mobility needs to be assessed carefully to distinguish between peri-implant tissue destruction due to loss of osseointegration and peri-implant mucositis due to failing (mobile or fractured) prosthetic components (Fig. 11.2a, b).

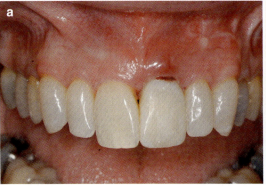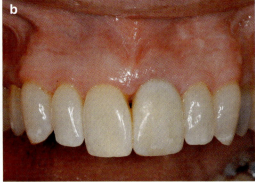

Fig. 11.2 (a) Peri-implant mucositis as a result of micro-movement due to inadequately tightened abutment screw (maxillary left central incisor). (b) Uneventful healing 2 weeks following adequate torque of abutment screw

However, significant amounts of peri-implant bone loss may not be detected with either of these methods due to their low sensitivity. Both methods might, however, be helpful in determining initial implant stability at the time of implant placement to assist in selecting the correct loading protocol.

Periodontal probing around dental implants provides important diagnostic information to evaluate peri-implant health and assist in long-term monitoring. Periodontal probing around dental implants does not seem to have a long-term effect on the soft tissue seal, since complete epithelial reattachment will occur within 5 days following probing with no signs of residual soft tissue damage. Traditionally the use of plastic periodontal probes has been recommended even though conventional metal probes do not appear to elicit any adverse effects on the implant surface or surrounding tissues. When considering probing as a test method, the difference between peri-implant probing and periodontal probing around healthy teeth must be understood. Specifically, the peri-implant probing depth typically measures the thickness of the surrounding sulcus, junctional epithelium, and connective tissue attachment and correlates, therefore, more closely with the level of the surrounding bone than the apical termination of the junctional epithelium (aJE) around dental implants. With probing around healthy teeth, the probing will generally be limited by the connective tissue fiber bundles that insert into the cementum lining the tooth root (See Chapter 1, Figure 1.5 a,b). Dental implants placed at bone level might therefore exhibit probing depths slightly greater than 4 mm at baseline (delivery of final implant-supported restoration). Increases in clinical probing depth over time, however, are usually associated with progressive loss of clinical attachment including peri-implant bone and should therefore be viewed as a sign of peri-implant disease.

It is generally believed that periodontal pathogens that cause periodontitis are also related to the onset and progression of peri-implant disease. Several microbiological tests are commercially available to measure the levels of putative periodontal pathogens either in saliva samples or

through paper-point sampling from peri-implant pockets. It might, therefore, be prudent to measure spirochetes and Gram-negative mobile anaerobic bacteria levels in patients with signs of peri-implantitis to better assist in selecting appropriate treatment options.

Etiology of Biological Complications Due to Residual Excess Cement

As discussed previously in this book, bacterial colonization, foreign body reaction, corrosive effects, and allergic reactions might play a role in the etiopathogenesis of biological complications due to residual excess cement. Different luting cements exhibit varying degrees of bacterial protection against periodontal pathogens due to their inherent antibacterial activities and solubility patterns. It is also known that some luting cements might elicit significant inflammatory responses and cytotoxicity in conjunction with foreign body reactions presenting as multinucleated giant cells. Additionally, micro-movement of loose cement particles might play a role in causing biological complications around dental implants similar to mobile prosthetic components (seen in Fig. 11.2a, b) that cause peri-implant mucositis if not detected early.

Treatment Modalities

Implant success is defined as implants with no pain, mobility, or radiolucencies and no more than 0.2 mm of peri-implant bone loss annually following the first year of loading. Additionally, peri-implant hard and soft tissues should remain healthy, and the patient should be satisfied with the final result both from esthetic and functional point of view. Biological complications are one of many etiologic factors for implant failures and involve pathologic changes in the peri-implant hard and soft tissues. Inflammatory changes in response to residual excess cement (REC) are prevalent and present a therapeutic challenge in maintaining healthy peri-implant tissues. The following paragraphs will discuss several treatment modalities that will aim at removing the foreign etiologic agent (REC) and help in preserving or restoring lost peri-implant soft and hard tissue structures utilizing an incremental therapeutic approach.

While biological complications associated with residual excess cement can be due to bacterial colonization, foreign body, corrosion effects, and/or allergic reactions, removing contaminants from the implant surface and surrounding tissues is considered the most important step during surgical management.

Decontamination of the Implant Surface

Many different decontamination techniques including mechanical, chemical, and electrochemical disinfection have been studied in the past. Ultrasonic scalers, plastic-tip scalers, titanium curettes, air-powder systems, rubber cups, titanium brushes, and cotton pellets have been used in combination with various chemicals including chlorhexidine solution or gel, stannous fluoride, tetracycline, minocycline, citric acid, hydrogen peroxide, and saline to decontaminate the implant surface. Photodynamic therapy, as well as different types of laser, including Er:YAG, Nd:YAG, and CO_2 lasers, have been tested in animals and clinical settings. More recently, electrochemical disinfection of dental implants using electrolysis to remove adherent bacteria from the implant surface is showing promising results as a method to decontaminate dental implants. While most of these decontamination methods have shown efficacy at removing biofilms, attempts to compare different decontamination methods have failed to show significant differences in treatment outcome.

Removal of residual excess cement requires mechanical debridement of the implant surface with either hand- or power-driven devices and depends significantly on the morphology of the peri-implant defect. A recent study indicates that implants surrounded by bony walls are less accessible for mechanical debridement even when air-flow devices are used. Clinicians currently use glycine-based air-flow devices as well as chemicals, including chlorhexidine and tetracycline solutions, to decontaminate the implant surface. It is still not clear if decontaminating implant surfaces will result in re-osseointegration of the entire implant. Even pristine implants placed into artificially created peri-implant defects show significantly less bone to implant contact as the width of the gap increased. Although some animal studies have shown the possibility of re-osseointegration of previously contaminated implant surfaces, achievement of re-osseointegration in a clinical setting might still be elusive. The therapeutic goal is the preparation of an implant surface that is biologically compatible with the peri-implant tissues and no signs of inflammation such as swelling, bleeding, or suppuration.

Nonsurgical Approach to Remove REC

"Less is more," a phrase coined by Robert Browning (1855), still holds true for many procedures in clinical dentistry today. Generally, provided the goal of therapy is achieved, the less invasive the intervention, the more postoperative comfort for the patient, and the faster the healing occurs. The less the mucoperiosteal flaps need to be elevated, the more the mucogingival architecture will be preserved. The following case history (Fig. 11.3a–g) demonstrates a clinical example of residual excess cement causing peri-implant mucositis that was subsequently treated utilizing the least invasive approach possible. The immediate implant was restored 12 weeks following

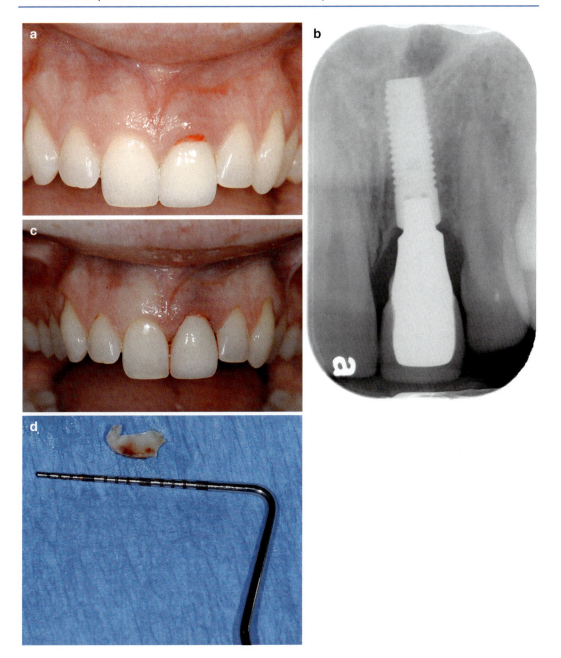

Fig. 11.3 (**a**) Clinical example of residual excess cement causing peri-implant mucositis (maxillary left central incisor). (**b**) Radiograph with typical "peripheral eggshell" effect indicating residual excess cement at crown/abutment margin. (**c**) Status post removal of residual excess cement; (**d**) excess cement removed. (**e**) Radiographic evaluation following cement removal indicating lack of REC; (**f**) 2 weeks later. (**g**) Uneventful healing 4 months following removal of REC

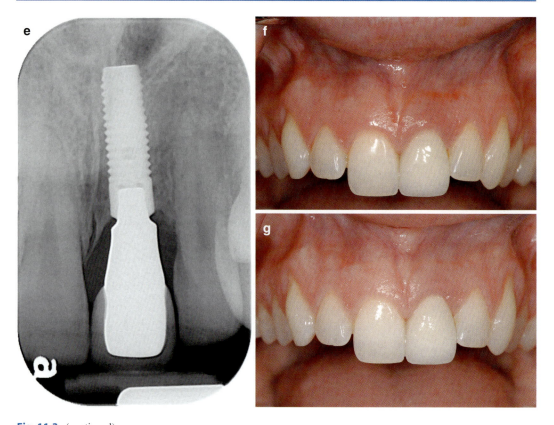

Fig. 11.3 (continued)

implantation with a zirconia computer-aided design-computer-aided manufactured (CAD-CAM) abutment, utilizing temporary luting cement (TempBond, Kerr). The patient presented two years following restoration with signs of peri-implant mucositis in combination with tenderness to palpation of the peri-implant soft tissues (Fig. 11.3a). A typical "peripheral eggshell effect" was evident upon radiographic examination, confirming the diagnosis of REC (Fig. 11.3b). Additionally, no radiographic bone loss could be detected ruling out the diagnosis of peri-implantitis. The treatment consisted of meticulous cement removal utilizing hand instruments and piezoelectric devices followed by copious irrigation with chlorhexidine gluconate solution and digital pressure to achieve adequate hemostasis postoperatively (Fig. 11.3c, d).

Uneventful healing was evident at 2 weeks, and complete resolution of the soft tissue defect was observed 4 months following therapeutic intervention (Fig. 11.3e–g). Subgingival debridement, including removal of excess luting cement, traditionally entails the use of plastic curettes and polishing pastes. Most plastic instruments, however, are highly flexible and can therefore not be used to dislodge subgingival calculus and dental cements with high bond strengths. Additionally, those instruments carry an increased risk of leaving remnants of the instrument material in the surgical site, compromising the wound healing. Stainless steel hand instruments, on the other hand, might leave significant damage on the treated implant surface, with subsequent increased plaque accumulation and biofilm growth. Titanium instruments are therefore considered state of the art to avoid the mentioned shortcomings, yet establishing a biocompatible implant surface after mechanical debridement.

Magnetostrictive or piezoelectric devices also seem to damage the implant surface if conventional tips are used. Copper alloy or plastic-covered tips are believed to minimize the damaging effect on the implant surface but may also increase the risk of leaving material remnants behind. Irrespective of the instrument used, it seems to be a "conditio sine qua non" to remove the REC as thoroughly as possible to allow for soft tissue healing and "restitutio ad integrum." This should be accomplished even at the potential expense of damaging the implant surface, if necessary, since unequivocal evidence is missing to support the notion that a damaged implant surface will eventually lead to peri-implant mucositis or peri-implantitis.

Another, slightly more invasive, approach consists of removing the entire cemented implant-supported restoration to obtain extraoral access for cement removal; this treatment modality is mainly indicated in the esthetic zone to avoid negative esthetic sequelae following surgical intervention.

Case Report (Fig. 11.4a–e) A female patient 45 years of age had an implant placed several years earlier. She presented complaining of inflammation around the implant site. A radiograph did not indicate REC presence; however, this is not uncommon as described in the previous chapters within this book. REC was suspected due to the depth of the restorative margin, so a procedure designed to evaluate the site was proposed to and accepted by the patient. Initially the crown/abutment complex would have to be removed. To obtain access to the contaminated abutment, a hole was prepared through the implant-supported crown to access the implant-abutment screw. The crown and abutment were removed by counter-torquing the abutment screw (Fig. 11.4b, c). Residual excess cement was present as suspected. The foreign material was carefully removed, and the site cleaned with chlorhexidine gluconate solution. The crown/abutment complex was also cleaned then retightened to the recommended torque and the screw access site within the crown restored with composite, thereby converting a cement-retained restoration into a screw-retained

restoration. Significant resolution of the peri-implant mucositis was observed 6 weeks following treatment (Fig. 11.4d). Subsequently, a more appropriately designed abutment with a more coronally placed cement margin and a new crown were made and delivered. Ten months after the initial visit, the implant restoration remained clinically inflammation free (Fig. 11.4e) with complete resolution.

Surgical Approach to Remove Residual Excess Cement (REC)

The advantage of a noninvasive approach to remove REC is evident, especially in situations that are esthetically challenging, and adequate access for cement removal is likely, for example the maxillary anterior zone. In situations, however, where complete cement removal cannot be accomplished utilizing a closed-flap approach, surgical intervention becomes more appropriate. Raising soft tissue flaps to allow access to the site may also be combined with antimicrobial therapy, regenerative techniques, or adjunctive laser therapy. Along with an improvement to access the implant body for debridement, the soft tissues may also be surgically accessed allowing removal of any foreign body matter that may also be present.

Most of the surgical techniques employed to treat peri-implantitis as a result of REC have been derived from and used successfully to treat periodontal lesions around natural teeth. Access flap, removal of granulation and/or granulomatous tissue, and surface decontamination are a common practice in treating periodontal or peri-implant defects.

A clinical example demonstrating the effectiveness of open flap debridement is provided in the following case example: A 72-year-old male in good health had 2 implants placed in a one-stage surgical procedure, with healing caps, in the maxillary first and second premolar sites. After allowing for a healing period of 4 months, the implants were deemed sufficiently osseointegrated to allow for final restoration and the treatment completed. After restoration, the first annual

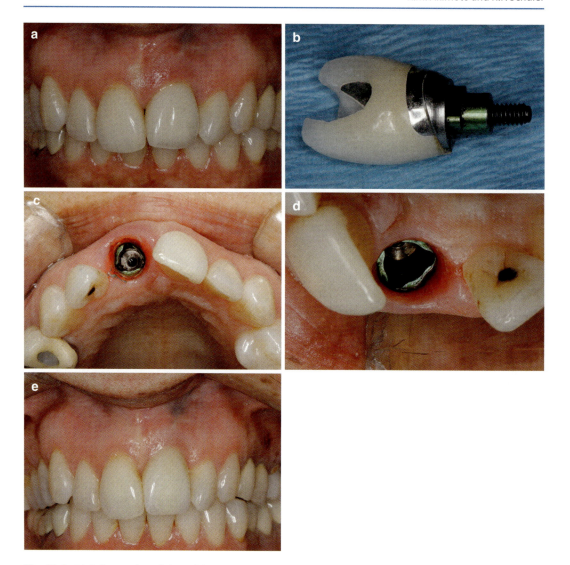

Fig. 11.4 (**a**) Inflammation of the peri-implant mucosa. Residual cement was not detected on radiographic survey. However, considering the restorative design with a deep cement margin, incomplete removal of cement was suspected. (**b**) The decision was made to remove the crown and the abutment, by creating an access to the abutment screw. Upon removal of the crown/abutment complex, residual cement was found. Seen here in the distal- buccal aspect of the sulcus. (**c**) Occlusal view immediately after removal of the crown. Inflammation is found at the sulcus. (**d**) Six weeks after removal of cement. Upon removal of the crown/abutment complex, absence of inflammation was found. (**e**) Facial view 10 months after the initial visit. The crown and abutment were remade

recall appointment revealed no issues. However at the second annual patient follow-up examination, intraoral radiographs revealed REC on both implants (Fig. 11.5a, b). The time line prior to discovering any issues appears to corroborate Wilson's study, which found a delay of between 4 months and nearly 9.5 years, with a mean of 3 years, before any issue with the implant is found when cement is involved in the pathogenesis of peri-implant disease.

Local anesthesia was obtained and a full-thickness flap was elevated to allow for adequate visualization of the peri-implant defects. The mucogingival flap was designed to preserve as much keratinized tissue as possible and allow for adequate visual inspection (Fig. 11.5c). Excess

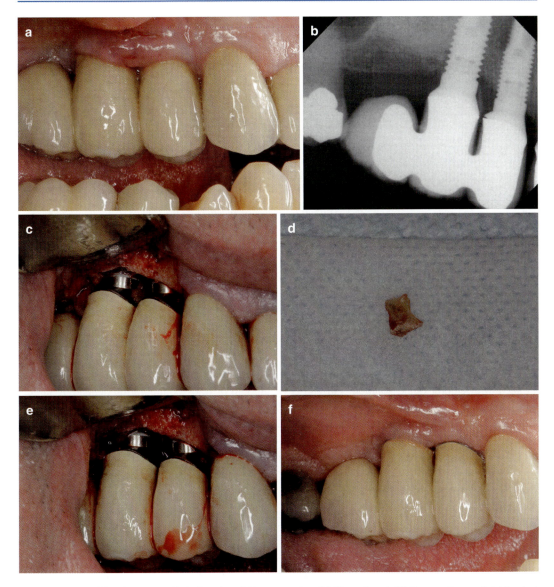

Fig. 11.5 (**a**) Peri-implant mucositis is found on follow-up exam after the restoration was completed. (**b**) Radiograph of the area indicates REC. (**c**) Upon flap ele-vation, REC was found. (**d**) Removed cement. (**e**) Implant site following cement removal. (**f**) Uneventful healing 3 months post treatment

cement was identified and removed followed by implant surface decontamination (Fig. 11.5d, e) using hand instruments and piezoelectric devices. The mucoperiosteal flap was then apically positioned allowing for primary closure utilizing 6-0 polypropylene sutures. Complete resolution of the peri-implant mucositis resulted within three months following surgical intervention (Fig. 11.5f).

The use of implant debridement instruments made of titanium bristles with a stainless steel shaft is particularly favorable in achieving a "clean" implant surface following debridement of the contaminated implant surface with conventional instruments (Straumann guide manual). A conventional surgical or oscillating (maximum of 900 oscillations per minute (OPM) handpiece may be used with the brush attachment. The following case

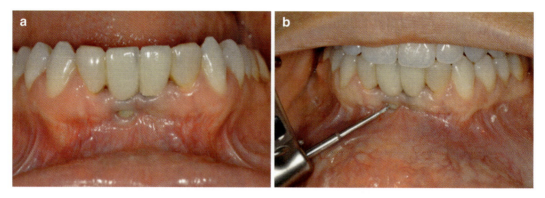

Fig. 11.6 (**a**, **b**) Use of titanium brush through a soft tissue fenestration to clean the implant site

report describes the use of the titanium brush (Fig. 11.6a, b). In this particular situation direct access was available through the soft tissue fenestration that existed, so no surgical flap was required. Debridement was carried out using the titanium brush on a conventional handpiece (Salvin). The site was carefully evaluated to confirm all undesirable material on the implant had been removed and cleaned with chlorhexidine solution. An autogenous soft tissue graft derived from the palatal tissue was used to cover the mucosal fenestration in order to achieve complete coverage of the formerly exposed and contaminated implant surface.

Surgical Approach to Remove REC in Combination with Regenerative Techniques

In the presence of more advanced peri-implant bone loss and crater-like defects, regenerative techniques might be employed. Schwartz classified peri-implant bony defects as they relate to morphologies that are amenable to hard tissue augmentation.

Class I Well defined intra-bony peri-implant defects that may present 3- or 4- wall defects or bony dehiscence. These have some ability to retain and support bone graft materials.

Class 2 Represents a more horizontal bone loss pattern.

The better the peri-implant bony defect is capable of retaining and supporting the bone graft, the more bone regeneration and clinical attachment gain will be achieved following surgi-

cal regenerative therapy. The use of bone graft material in combination with regenerative membranes might be considered in severe 3-wall defects. The possibility of re-osseointegration at contaminated implant surfaces was reviewed by Renvert et al. They concluded based on animal studies that re-osseointegration is not possible for the entire contaminated implant surface, with the amount of re-osseointegration depending largely on the implant surface and type of access surgery selected.

Surgical intervention with or without concomitant regenerative procedures carries the risk of esthetic complications including exposure of implant components and loss of peri-implant soft tissues.

Case Report A female patient in good health presented with a complete horizontal fracture of an maxillary left left lateral incisor. Options for treatment included extraction of the root and replacement with a fixed conventional tooth-borne bridge or an implant, as the root was considered too short for endodontic therapy and post core placement. The patient had experience with dental implants as the contralateral site was previously replaced with a dental implant and restoration (Fig. 11.7a–h).

The patient opted for extraction, and an immediate implant was placed (Fig. 11.7a). A radiograph was made to show the final implant placement (Fig. 11.7b). A custom healing abutment was fabricated and placed at the time of implant placement, and the site was allowed to heal for 3 months. Once clinical osseointegration was confirmed by the implant surgeon, the patient was referred back to the restorative dentist for completion of treatment.

Four-and-a-half years after the final cemented crown was placed, the patient returned to the implant surgeon complaining of pain and swelling (Fig. 11.7c). Radiographic examination indicated evidence of significant bone loss associated with the implant (Fig. 11.7d).

A full-thickness surgical flap was elevated, revealing a large bony dehiscence and black discolored mass of foreign material on the implant surface (Fig. 11.7e). Further evaluation determined the mass to consist of REC with the discoloration

a result of hemosiderin staining from blood breakdown products. The mass was removed and the site cleaned first using hand instrumentation then air abrasion (Fig. 11.7f). Demineralized bovine bone matrix was grafted and covered with a resorbable collagen membrane and the surgical site closed and sutured (Fig. 11.7g).

The esthetic outcome is unlikely to be acceptable for many patients even if a complete resolution of the inflammatory process is achieved (Fig. 11.7h). Explantation of the affected implant followed by regenerative therapy and reimplantation might therefore be considered as an alternative treatment modality to achieve a more favorable esthetic outcome.

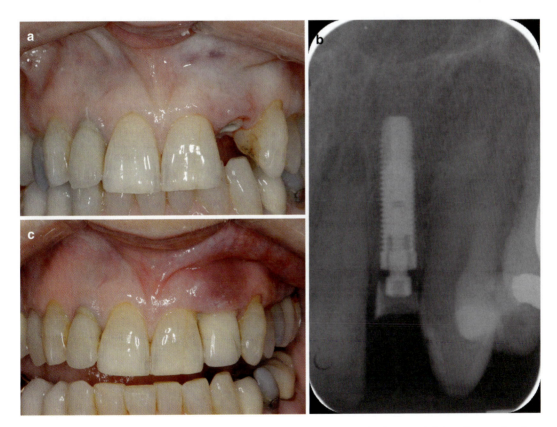

Fig. 11.7 (**a**) Tooth #10 was removed and immediate implant was placed with customized healing abutment. Clinical view 3 months after the surgery, immediately prior to the restorative procedure. (**b**) Radiograph of the area showing good peri-implant bone level. (**c**) Four-and-a-half years after restoration, patient presented with severe gingival inflammation. (**d**) Radiograph of the area shows significant peri-implant bone loss. (**e**) Upon flap elevation, large amounts of foreign material deposits were found on implant surface. (**f**) Air-powder spray device was used to clean implant surface. Note deep cement margin on the abutment. (**g**) Demineralized bovine bone matrix was grafted and covered with collagen membrane. (**h**) Two months post-op (Note significant loss of soft tissue around the implant)

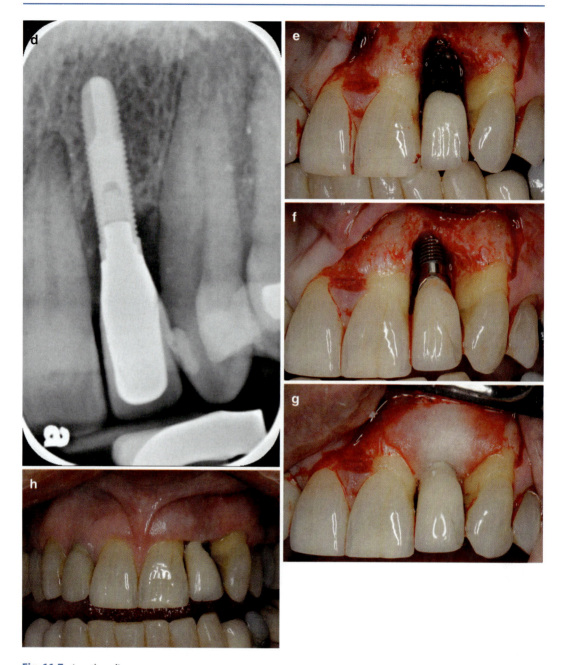

Fig. 11.7 (continued)

Long-Term Outcome Following Surgical Regenerative Therapy

Case Report A female patient 47 years of age presented for extraction of the maxillary right canine due to secondary caries resulting from repair of an external resorption lesion. The tooth had been diagnosed with irreversible pulpitis, and treatment options were provided to the patient. These included root canal therapy and clinical crown lengthening with possible post core crown preparation (due to the extent of the lesion) or replacement of the tooth with a dental implant (Fig. 11.8a, b). The patient opted to have

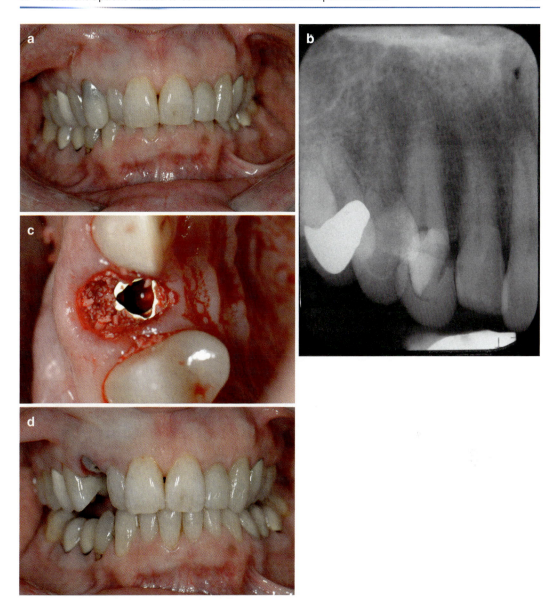

Fig. 11.8 (**a**) Maxillary right canine with extensive secondary caries. Clinical view at the time of initial presentation. (**b**) Initial radiograph. Note note extensive caries under the existing restoration. (**c**) The tooth was removed and implant was placed immediately into the extraction socket. The remaining gap facial to the implant was grafted with deproteinized bovine bone mineral (DBBM). (**d**) Customized healing abutment was fabricated. Clinical view immediately after the procedure. (**e**) Radiograph 3 months post-implant placement upon confirmation of the integration. (**f**) Clinical view 3 years after implant was restored. Swelling is seen around the implant. (**g**) Radiograph shows significant peri-implant bone loss. (**h**) Clinical view upon flap reflection. Note residual cement (REC) with peri-implant bone loss. (**i**) Clinical view after removal of the deposits and decontamination. (**j**) Clinical view with deproteinized bovine bone mineral (DBBM) in place. (**k**) Surgical site closed and sutures placed. (**l**) Clinical view 5 years post decontamination and surgical repair. Surgical repair site failed to fully resolve. Bleeding with suppuration were present on probing. (**m**) Radiograph taken at 5-year follow-up

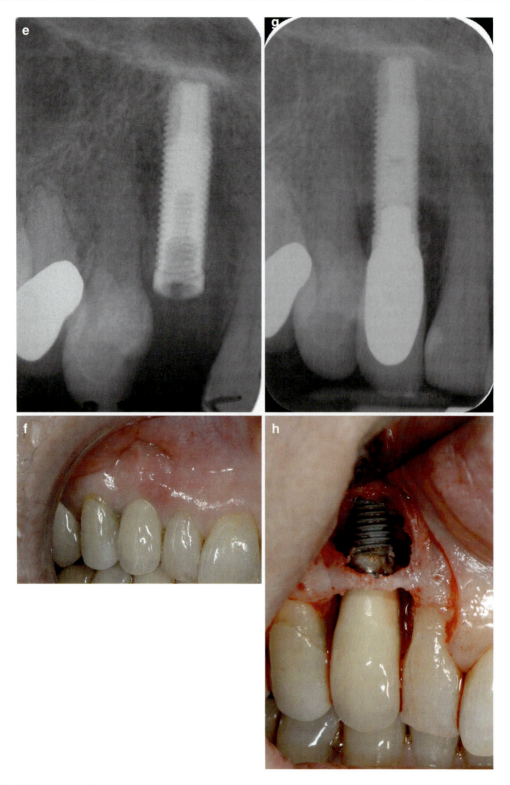

Fig. 11.8 (continued)

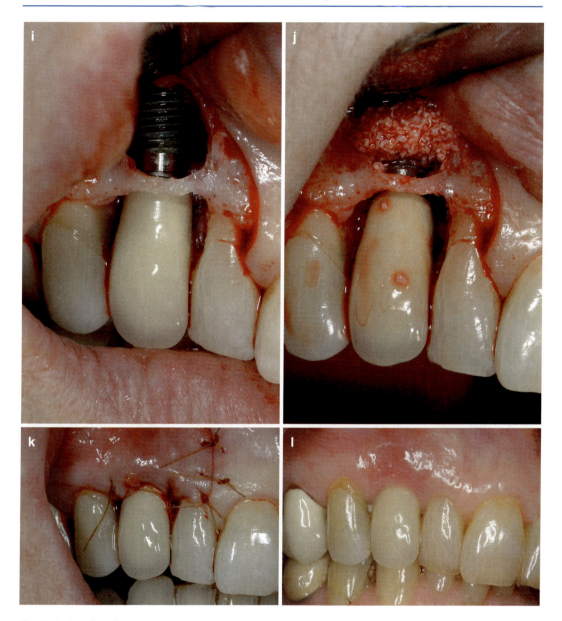

Fig. 11.8 (continued)

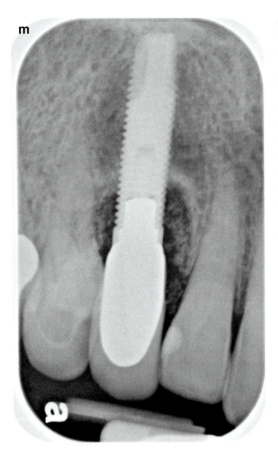

m

Fig. 11.8 (continued)

the tooth removed. At the time of extraction, the site was evaluated and measured to see if it was possible to use an immediate implant placement protocol. The extraction socket was intact, and an immediate implant placed (Fig. 11.8c, d). Integration of the implant was confirmed several months later both clinically and radiographically (Fig. 11.8e), and the patient returned to the restorative dentist for restoration with a cement-retained implant-supported crown.

Three years later, the patient presented at the periodontist's office with significant swelling around the implant and complaining of tenderness on palpation of the site (Fig. 11.8f). Radiographic evaluation revealed excessive peri-implant bone loss in combination with REC (Fig. 11.8g). Upon flap reflection, residual cement was found surrounding the implant-abutment interface resulting

in a significant amount of peri-implant bone loss including the partial loss of the buccal plate (Fig. 11.8h). An air-flow device was used to remove all deposits on the implant surface followed by copious irrigation with 0.12 % chlorhexidine gluconate in an attempt to decontaminate the implant surface (Fig. 11.8i). To cover the implant initially, deproteinized bovine bone mineral (DBBM) was placed against the cleansed surface, and then a bovine-derived collagen membrane was used. To complete the graft procedure (Fig. 11.8j), flap adaptation was performed, and closure was achieved with 6-0 gut sutures (Fig. 11.8k). Systemic antibiotics (amoxicillin) were then prescribed for 10 days and combined with chlorhexidine gluconate rinses twice daily for 2 weeks.

Although an attempt was made to resolve the peri-implant disease with surgical intervention, the inflammation remained and resolution did not occur. This was evident at subsequent follow-up visits (Fig. 11.8l, m). Suppuration and bleeding were found upon probing, and while the implant survived during this period, surgical intervention clearly failed to re-establish healthy peri-implant tissues. This problem is not uncommon with Schwartz reporting poor surgical outcomes associated with bony dehiscences. When this type of defect is found in the esthetic zone, it may be better to remove the implant rather than trying to regenerate the peri-implant tissues.

Explantation and Subsequent Implant Replacement

Explanation therapy is indicated in situations where previous regenerative attempts were unsuccessful or when peri-implant bone loss exceeds more than 50 % of the implant surface. Class I peri-implant defects tend to yield better results compared to class II (characterized by consistent horizontal bone loss by Schwarz) defects in their inherent regenerative potential following removal of the failing dental implant. Different implant removal systems are available (Implant Extraction System, Biotechnology

Institute, Blue Bell, PA, USA) to remove failing implants minimizing the need for bone trephination, which would leave larger circumferential bone defects. The atraumatic extraction systems are counter-threaded which are inserted directly into the implant in a counterclockwise manner. The torque wrench is subsequently fitted and further turned counterclockwise with up to 200 Ncm until the osseointegration between the implant and surrounding bone fails, releasing the implant. In the event that the counter-torque exceeds 200 Ncm and the implant fails to unscrew, a trephine bur is recommended to remove the most coronal 3–4 mm of the bone from the implant (BTI manual). This approach facilitates rapid and predictable implant removal with minimal trauma to the peri-implant bone and tissues.

Case Presentation (Fig. 11.9a–g) A male patient presented with a failing implant in the mandibular right second premolar region location as evidenced by increased peri-implant

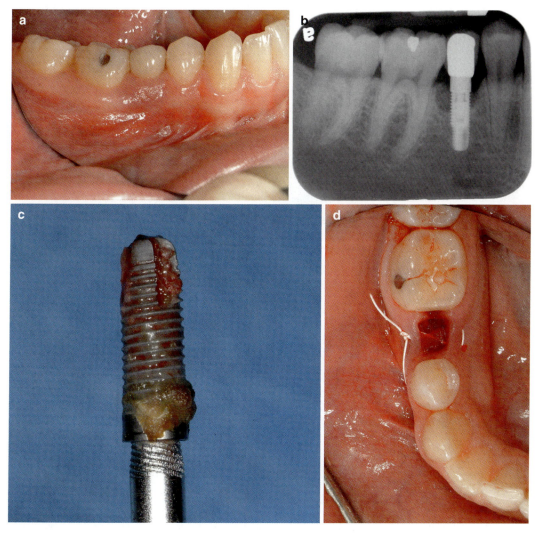

Fig. 11.9 (a) Clinical photograph and (b) radiographic image of implant site. Lower right second premolar presenting with signs of peri-implantitis. (c) Implant removal using counter-torque device seen within the implant. REC is seen at the implant collar. (d) The explanted implant site is cleaned and graft material placed. (e) New implant placement with healing cap in situ. (f) Subsequent new restoration with screw-retained crown 3 months later. (g) Final radiographs demonstrating adequate peri-implant bone levels (Photo courtesy of Dr. Darrin Rapoport)

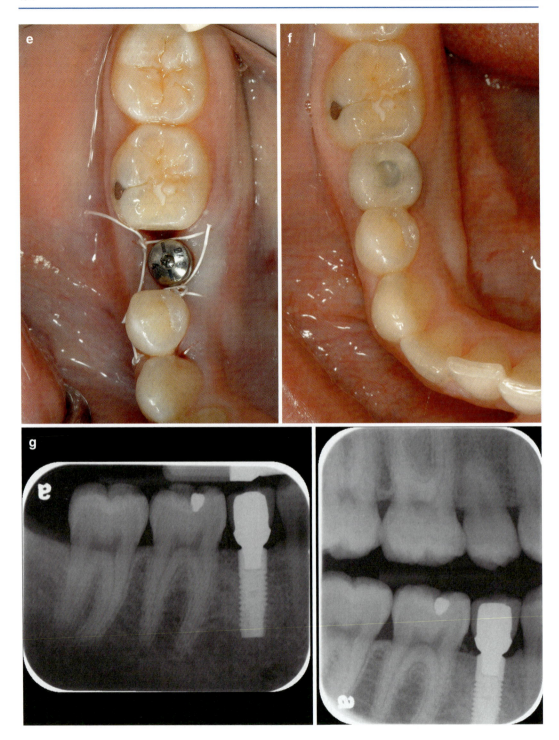

Fig. 11.9 (continued)

probing depth in combination with suppuration and severe radiographic peri-implant bone loss. His dental history revealed previous attempts to save the failing implant via nonsurgical and surgical means including regenerative procedures. Findings, treatment options, risks, and benefits were reviewed with the patient, and the need for implant removal was explained. The implant was subsequently removed with the use of an atraumatic extraction system, and its explantation site was grafted with rehydrated solvent-dehydrated allograft (SDA) and covered with a collagen membrane. Surgical field closure with good hemostasis was accomplished with 5-0 ePTFE sutures. The site was left for 4 months of healing prior to implant replacement. A replacement implant was subsequently placed and a further 3 months of healing to allow for osseointegration before the implant was restored, this time with a screw-retained implant-supported restoration thereby avoiding the need for any type of luting cement.

Conclusion

Residual excess cement is one of many etiologic factors for the development of peri-implant mucositis, peri-implantitis, and possible loss of osseointegration of dental implants. The use of screw-retained implant-supported restorations would eliminate the need for luting cements and therefore eliminate a potential component cause for implant failures. Unfortunately, anatomical, esthetic, and occlusal considerations might require the use of cement-retained, implant-supported restorations.

This chapter proposes an incremental treatment approach to prevent or treat peri-implant mucositis and/or peri-implantitis related to residual excess cement (see Fig. 11.10). A less invasive treatment approach is always preferable to minimize postoperative morbidity and avoid negative esthetic sequels. In certain clinical indications, removal of the failing implant might be the treatment modality of choice in order to avoid additional damage to the peri-implant structures or adjacent periodontia.

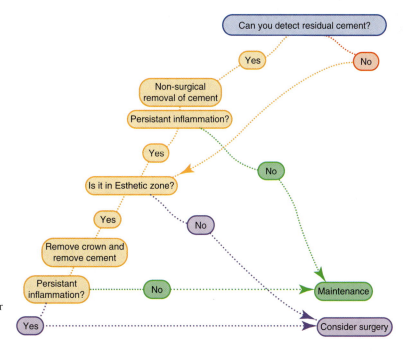

Fig. 11.10 Proposed incremental treatment approach to prevent or treat peri-implant mucositis and/or peri-implantitis related to residual excess cement

Bibliography

Adell R, Lekhol U, Rockler B, Branemark PI. A 15-year study of osseointegrated implants in the treatment of the edentulous jaw. Int J Oral Surg. 1981;10: 387–416.

Akimoto K, Becker W, Persson R, Baker DA, Rohrer MD, O'Neal RB. Evaluation of titanium implants placed into simulated extraction sockets: a study in dogs. Int J Oral Maxillofac Implants. 1999;14:351–60.

Albrektsson T, Jansson T, Lekholm U. Osseointegrated dental implants. Dent Clin North Am. 1986;30: 151–74.

Atassi F. Periimplant probing: positives and negatives. Implant Dent. 2002;11:356–62.

Balleri P, Cozzolino A, Ghelli L, Momicchioli G, Varriale A. Stability measurements of osseointegrated implants using Osstell in partially edentulous jaws after 1 year of loading: a pilot study. Clin Implant Dent Relat Res. 2002;4:128–32.

Becker W, Becker BE, Berg L, Samsam C. Clinical and volumetric analysis of three-wall intrabony defects following open flap debridement. J Periodontol. 1986;57:277–85.

Cavusoglu Y, Sahin E, Akca K. Efficacy of resonance frequency analysis in the diagnosis of compromised bone-implant interface. Implant Dent. 2012;21: 394–8.

Corbella S, Del Fabbro M, Taschieri S, De Siena F, Francetti L. Clinical evaluation of an implant maintenance protocol for the prevention of peri-implant diseases in patients treated with immediately loaded full-arch rehabilitations. Int J Dent Hyg. 2011;9: 216–22.

de Waal YC, Raghoebar GM, Huddleston Slater JJ, Meijer HJ, Winkel EG, van Winkelhoff AJ. Implant decontamination during surgical peri-implantitis treatment: a randomized, double-blind, placebo-controlled trial. J Clin Periodontol. 2013;40:186–95.

Etter TH, Hakanson I, Lang NP, Trejo PM, Caffesse RG. Healing after standardized clinical probing of the perlimplant soft tissue seal: a histomorphometric study in dogs. Clin Oral Implants Res. 2002;13: 571–80.

Gerber J, Wenaweser D, Heitz-Mayfield L, Lang NP, Persson GR. Comparison of bacterial plaque samples from titanium implant and tooth surfaces by different methods. Clin Oral Implants Res. 2006;17:1–7.

Heitz-Mayfield LJ. Diagnosis and management of peri-implant diseases. Aust Dent J. 2008;53 Suppl 1: S43–8.

Ito T, Yasuda M, Kaneko H, Sasaki H, Kato T, Yajima Y. Clinical evaluation of salivary periodontal pathogen levels by real-time polymerase chain reaction in patients before dental implant treatment. Clin Oral Implants Res. 2014;25(8):977–82.

Kawashima H, Sato S, Kishida M, Yagi H, Matsumoto K, Ito K. Treatment of titanium dental implants with three piezoelectric ultrasonic scalers: an in vivo study. J Periodontol. 2007;78:1689–94.

Kolonidis SG, Renvert S, Hammerle CH, Lang NP, Harris D, Claffey N. Osseointegration on implant surfaces previously contaminated with plaque. An experimental study in the dog. Clin Oral Implants Res. 2003;14:373–80.

Korkmaz FM, Tuzuner T, Baygin O, Buruk CK, Durkan R, Bagis B. Antibacterial activity, surface roughness, flexural strength, and solubility of conventional luting cements containing chlorhexidine diacetate/cetrimide mixtures. J Prosthet Dent. 2013;110:107–15.

Lindhe J, Meyle J. Peri-implant diseases: Consensus Report of the Sixth European Workshop on Periodontology. J Clin Periodontol. 2008;35:282–5.

Mohn D, Zehnder M, Stark WJ, Imfeld T. Electrochemical disinfection of dental implants–a proof of concept. PLoS One. 2011;6:e16157.

Mombelli A. Microbiology and antimicrobial therapy of peri-implantitis. Periodontol 2000. 2002;28:177–89.

Olive J, Aparicio C. Periotest method as a measure of osseointegrated oral implant stability. Int J Oral Maxillofac Implants. 1990;5:390–400.

Persson LG, Araujo MG, Berglundh T, Grondahl K, Lindhe J. Resolution of peri-implantitis following treatment. An experimental study in the dog. Clin Oral Implants Res. 1999;10:195–203.

Renvert S, Polyzois I, Maguire R. Re-osseointegration on previously contaminated surfaces: a systematic review. Clin Oral Implants Res. 2009;20 Suppl 4:216–27.

Rosenberg ES, Torosian JP, Slots J. Microbial differences in 2 clinically distinct types of failures of osseointegrated implants. Clin Oral Implants Res. 1991;2:135–44.

Sahrmann P, Ronay V, Sener B, Jung RE, Attin T, Schmidlin PR. Cleaning potential of glycine air-flow application in an in vitro peri-implantitis model. Clin Oral Implants Res. 2013;24:666–70.

Schou S, Holmstrup P, Jorgensen T, Skovgaard LT, Stoltze K, Hjørting-Hansen E, et al. Implant surface preparation in the surgical treatment of experimental peri-implantitis with autogenous bone graft and ePTFE membrane in cynomolgus monkeys. Clin Oral Implants Res. 2003;14:412–22.

Schwarz F, Sahm N, Schwarz K, Becker J. Impact of defect configuration on the clinical outcome following surgical regenerative therapy of peri-implantitis. J Clin Periodontol. 2010a;37:449–55.

Schwarz F, Jung RE, Fienitz T, Wieland M, Becker J, Sager M. Impact of guided bone regeneration and defect dimension on wound healing at chemically modified hydrophilic titanium implant surfaces: an experimental study in dogs. J Clin Periodontol. 2010b;37:474–85.

Schwarz F, Sahm N, Iglhaut G, Becker J. Impact of the method of surface debridement and decontamination on the clinical outcome following combined surgical therapy of peri-implantitis: a randomized controlled clinical study. J Clin Periodontol. 2011;38:276–84.

Schwarz F, John G, Mainusch S, Sahm N, Becker J. Combined surgical therapy of peri-implantitis evaluating two methods of surface debridement and decontamination. A two-year clinical follow up report. J Clin Periodontol. 2012;39:789–97.

Sennerby L, Meredith N. Implant stability measurements using resonance frequency analysis: biological and biomechanical aspects and clinical implications. Periodontol 2000. 2008;47:51–66.

Shumaker ND, Metcalf BT, Toscano NT, Holtzclaw DJ. Periodontal and periimplant maintenance: a critical factor in long-term treatment success. Compend Contin Educ Dent. 2009;30:388–90, 392, 394.

Souza PP, Aranha AM, Hebling J, Giro EM, Costa CA. In vitro cytotoxicity and in vivo biocompatibility of contemporary resin-modified glass-ionomer cements. Dent Mater. 2006;22:838–44.

Subramani K, Wismeijer D. Decontamination of titanium implant surface and re-osseointegration to treat peri-implantitis: a literature review. Int J Oral Maxillofac Implants. 2012;27:1043–54.

Vervaeke S, Collaert B, Cosyn J, Deschepper E, De Bruyn H. A multifactorial analysis to identify predictors of implant failure and peri-implant bone loss. Clin Implant Dent Relat Res. 2013. doi:10.1111/cid.12149.

Wadhwani CP, Chung KH. The role of cements in dental implant success, Part 2. Dent Today. 2013;32(46): 48–51.

Wadhwani CP, Schwedhelm ER. The role of cements in dental implant success, Part I. Dent Today. 2013; 32:74–8; quiz 78–9.

Wilson Jr TG. The positive relationship between excess cement and peri-implant disease: a prospective clinical endoscopic study. J Periodontol. 2009;80:1388–92.

Index

C.P.K. Wadhwani (ed.), *Cementation in Dental Implantology: An Evidence-Based Guide*,
DOI 10.1007/978-3-642-55163-51, © Springer-Verlag Berlin Heidelberg 2015